AutPlay® Therapy Play and Social Groups

The second edition of *AutPlay® Therapy Play and Social Groups* provides a neurodiversity-affirming perspective to help children and parents build healthy relationships, gain positive identity, build relationships with peers in ways that are meaningful for them, and help them navigate social situations to get what they want and need.

Practitioners are provided with a step-by-step guide for implementing play and social groups for neurodivergent children and adolescents. This unique group model incorporates the AutPlay Therapy framework focused on neurodiversity-affirming methods, including the implementation of play therapy theory and approach. Updates to the second edition include a complete neurodiversity-affirming overhaul of the first five chapters, updated research and inclusive language, and a new chapter with more group interventions designed to address additional issues such as relationship building and connection.

Through this resource, practitioners across disciplines who work with neurodivergent children and adolescents will find a unique and valuable guide to implementing play and social-focused groups.

Robert Jason Grant is the creator of AutPlay® Therapy. He is a therapist, supervisor, and consultant and utilizes several years of advanced training and his own lived neurodivergent experience to provide affirming services to children and their families.

Tracy Turner-Bumberry is a licensed professional counsellor and registered play therapist who operates a private practice in Macon, Georgia. She is also a professional speaker and author.

AutPlay® Therapy Play and Social Groups

A Neurodiversity-Affirming Model
Second edition

Robert Jason Grant and
Tracy Turner-Bumberry

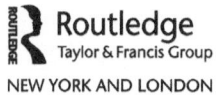

Routledge
Taylor & Francis Group
NEW YORK AND LONDON

Designed cover image: © Getty Images

Second edition published 2025
by Routledge
605 Third Avenue, New York, NY 10158

and by Routledge
4 Park Square, Milton Park, Abingdon, Oxon, OX14 4RN

Routledge is an imprint of the Taylor & Francis Group, an informa business

© 2025 Robert Jason Grant and Tracy Turner-Bumberry

The right of Robert Jason Grant and Tracy Turner-Bumberry
to be identified as authors of this work has been asserted in
accordance with sections 77 and 78 of the Copyright, Designs
and Patents Act 1988.

First edition published by Routledge 2021, *AutPlay® Therapy Play
and Social Skills Groups: A 10-Session Model*

ISBN: 9781032742489 (hbk)
ISBN: 9781032739144 (pbk)
ISBN: 9781003468370 (ebk)

DOI: 10.4324/9781003468370

Typeset in Times New Roman
by codeMantra

Contents

Acknowledgments

We would like to thank the colleagues who took time to review our book and provide us with feedback – Jessica Kitchens, Marshall Lyles, and Emily Kirchner-Morris. We would also like to thank Dr. Kevin Hull for his generous foreword.

Special acknowledgment to our families and friends who labored with us as we completed this book. Thank you for being patient and supportive.

Additionally, thank you to the neurodivergent community and all those who keep advocating, speaking, writing, and teaching for a neurodiversity-affirming society.

Foreword

"What should young people do with their lives today? Many things, obviously. But the most daring thing is to create stable communities in which the terrible disease of loneliness can be cured."

Kurt Vonnegut

A theme found in many neurodivergent individuals is the sense of being alone and misunderstood. The complications of neurodiversity can leave one feeling as if they exist in an isolated world. For many neurodivergent individuals, living in a neurotypically dominated world can be penetratingly painful, confusing, and frightening. As children navigate the stages of development, social situations and expectations become increasingly complicated. For neurodivergent young people who struggle with interpreting these situations and expectations, it can seem as though there are not only barriers but that the barriers are constantly shifting in size and shape. For the past twenty years, I have conducted group play therapy specifically for the neurodivergent population, and until recently, there were few resources available for practitioners like me. A quick survey of the resource landscape revealed even fewer resources that celebrated or affirmed the differences found in the neurodivergent, and many carried an agenda to fix or change the core self of the individual.

Robert Jason Grant and Tracey Turner-Bumberry have crafted an invaluable process to help neurodivergent children, adolescents, and families navigate and adapt to the social challenges that so often plague this population. *AutPlay Therapy Play and Social Groups: A Neurodiversity-Affirming Model (2nd Edition)* is beautifully written by two authors who display clinical mastery coupled with compassion. This volume is simple and direct and links information with technical approaches providing pathways for practitioners working with neurodivergent youth to experience social navigation and adaptation. The power of group interventions is highlighted in this text, but the focus goes far beyond the typical skill-based focus that has dominated the neurodivergent treatment landscape for many years. Instead, the authors keenly focus on attributes such as self-advocacy, building identity, and strengthening the parent-child relationship which is often ignored in most treatment modalities. The authors achieve an intricate balance between demonstrating the course for preparing the young person to be able to navigate and adapt to a neurotypical world, while preserving the core self and respecting key characteristics that make up who the child is. This is a testament to Dr. Grant and Turner-Bumberry's exceptional clinical understanding, balanced with empathy, and reflects their personal calling to work with this population.

I am pleased to present *AutPlay Therapy Play and Social Groups: A Neurodiversity-Affirming Model (2ⁿᵈ Edition)* as a unique gift to the world of practitioners who believe in the power of play, group process, and preserving the sacred self of neurodivergent individuals while increasing social flexibility and adaptation.

Kevin B. Hull,
PhD, Licensed Counselor,
Registered Play Therapist,
Certified Group Psychotherapist

Introduction

Neurodivergence and Social Navigation

Higashida (2013) explained that it is hard to believe anyone born as a human being really wants to be left alone and not have social contact. For neurodivergent individuals, it is not a lack of social contact that is the concern; it is the worry that they will encounter judgment and rejection from a neuronormative designed social expectation. This is why it can be challenging for neurodivergent people to be around other people (specifically neurotypical people), and thus they often end up navigating with other neurodivergent people or being by themselves where things are more predictable, clear, and less anxiety-producing.

Neurodivergent individuals do desire to have meaningful relationships and a realized social system, but because social situations are rarely affirming or accepting, the neurodivergent person can often find themselves in isolation. It's fairly understood that neurodivergent children can experience social navigation needs, and it's also understood that despite the possible needs, neurodivergent children do desire social connection. It is not about a lack of interest in social life; it's about a neuronormative culture that does not accept or value neurodivergent social navigation. This creates a myriad of challenging dynamics for the neurodivergent person – how to navigate a social system that the neurotypical population expects while also being your authentic neurodivergent self, how to avoid harmful constructs such as masking and camouflaging, how to advocate for changes in the way societal views social navigation, and how to find value and dignity in a world that views you as a deficit.

In the greater neurotypical society, most social understandings develop without formal instruction for neurotypical individuals, starting very early in life. Most children acquire the expected social understandings as part of their typical daily experiences and developmental growth. Many people cannot recall how they learned to look at someone when they were talking or exactly when they first learned to get in the back of the line and wait instead of pushing to the front. But somewhere these social understandings, along with many others, were learned and became part of their natural social navigation system. This is what it looks

DOI: 10.4324/9781003468370-1

and feels like to grow up neurotypical. These social understandings are not only learned very easily, but they also make sense, feel fine, and present no challenges to the person's identity. Because of this ease in social understandings, neurotypicals may not even realize that others struggle with these societal norms and be unaware of the difficulties neurodivergents face in society. This unawareness can lead to judgment and unrealistic expectations placed upon neurodivergents. This easy and natural social navigation process is not the same for neurodivergent individuals. What seems logical, typical, and easy to understand in neurotypical set standards does not always make sense or align with neurodivergent brains and operating systems. This might be fine if differences were accepted, valued, and appreciated; unfortunately, they are not. The neurodivergent way of social navigation is highly pathologized, judged through ableist ideology, and often results in harmful and traumatizing experiences for neurodivergent children.

Many people and systems demand a prescribed presentation and level of social functioning from neurodivergent children, and if it is not present, expect them to quickly address the "deficit" and begin to display the appropriate "social skills." In addition, it is often expected that the missing "social skills" should be taught, and the child will then be "normal." When this does not occur (as it never will with neurodivergent children), the child is often penalized and sometimes labeled as resistant or defiant. For neurodivergent children, a neurotypically expected "social skill" is not going to develop because an adult tells them to do it; these "social skills" are not going to become an understood part of the neurodivergent child's daily experience by punishing them when they do not display the expected social behavior. This is not how neurodiversity works. The neurodiversity paradigm, which states that diversity of neurotypes exists naturally across humans, requires a paradigm shift in the beliefs that have been held that social navigation must exist one way and any difference is a deficit that must be fixed.

Consider the following from Grant et al. (2022), which highlights the voice of autistic artist and writer Anastasia Phelps when sharing about her social experiences:

> *I like it when people talk to me like I am another human being like anyone else. I like it when they give me a chance instead of writing me off as a weirdo. Just like anyone else, I want acceptance, and I want to be listened to.*
>
> *I have had quite a few people talk to me like I am an infant. I have had former therapists address me in such tones, and even leaders and students from my church would talk to me in the same demeaning manner. The thing is, I know 90% of them don't necessarily do it with bad intent, however, that doesn't make it any less discouraging or hurtful to me.*
>
> *As a teen, I still struggle to insert myself in group conversations. I struggle to find openings where I can talk and yet not interrupt the others who wish to speak, or who may not have been finished. It really throws my mind into a frenzy.*

Oftentimes, especially among my peers, I just don't know how to express myself. I am conflicted on how to react socially, so I tend to watch rather than interact. Which sometimes results in me being perceived as stuck up or outlandish. The thing is, I can keep up with the conversation mentally, and as long as it is a topic I am familiar with, I can even join in. But I would rather not risk embarrassing myself socially if I can help it, since I already feel like everyone is already judging me.

Neurodivergent children often find the social functioning world confusing, frustrating, and sometimes scary. There is a great need for them to develop the ability to categorize and understand social systems in a way that makes sense to them and enables them to navigate the social situations in ways that honor their neurotype. For neurodivergent children to accomplish the social-related goals and experiences that are important to them, their desires and differences must be valued and supported by the people and systems with which they navigate. Koening (2012) proposed that social competency does not develop in isolation from cognitive, emotional, and other development. There is a continual interplay among these domains and competencies. When considering neurodivergent social navigation success, the whole child must be considered; otherwise, true sustainable awareness may not be fully realized, resulting in gaps in the child's self-concept and identity.

Implementing any social navigation intervention or approach requires the professional to see the whole child, not simply a child with particular "social skill struggles" or a child with a specific mental health diagnosis. Understanding a diagnosis and common features associated with a diagnosis is essential for being a prepared professional, but this should never replace or exclude the ability to see the fully developing neurodivergent child and respect the uniqueness of their spectrum of presentation.

Neurodivergent individuals can possess the same strengths and talents found in any neurotypical person, and they often possess unique strengths and abilities due to being neurodivergent. A neurodivergent child may have mental health needs related to social, emotional, relational, and other areas, and therapeutic intervention should focus on addressing these challenges. A growing amount of research is showing that neurodivergent individuals may benefit from unique strengths previously unnoticed by the general (neurotypical) population. Those involved and working with neurodivergent individuals should focus on each person and their individual areas of strength and growth, as well as the personality qualities that set them apart and make them unique. The more that is understood about how a neurodivergent child's brain is organized differently from a neurotypical brain, the more awareness is gained that a different way of organizing can be valued (Panzano, 2018).

Consider the following from Grant et al. (2022), which highlights the voice of autistic speaker and author Dr. Stephen Mark Shore discussing social experiences in one of his first employment settings:

I was closely supervised and was expected to fit in with all of the accountant/ business employees. The business uniform is the suit and tie… which drove me nuts. I can't stand to wear a tie. The only way I could survive was to ride my bicycle from where I lived (about 7 miles) to work and enjoy the out-of-doors for an hour and a half each day. It took 45 minutes to get to work this way as opposed to the 2 hours by public transportation. Made sense to me.

Riding my bicycle to work and changing into my suit in the basement of the office was too weird for them. The personnel officer told me that I had better take public transportation and arrive at the office in my suit. Thinking back to that time I realize that I could not have chosen a place that was more conservative, and conformist had I tried. Probably all financial institutions are like this. After a while I spent most of my time in their library reading business reference books as the supply of work seemed to dry up. On occasion, I would seek out work from other coworkers, or drop into one of the senior manager's office for a chat.

An assignment with a fellow accountant at the firm didn't work out well at all. I could never really understand what he wanted, and he seemed irritated at the things I did. The bank where we worked was overheated. In response to that I would often open the window and take off my shoes when I was sitting at the desk out of view of other people. He didn't like that at all. While auditing a ledger I mentioned to him that it was difficult to read some of the numbers.

One day the personnel officer called me into his office and told me he was letting me go. He said that I just didn't seem to fit in and suggested that there may have been a disability that I had failed to disclose to him when I interviewed for the job. That disability may very well have been there. To me, however, it was something of the past and it never occurred to me that accommodation may have been needed. I just thought I was stupid because I didn't "get it." Getting fired was very humiliating and embarrassing to me. With a fuzzy, heavy feeling in my head I gathered my belongings and left.

Grant et al. (2022) stated that neurodivergence does not have a singular look, feel, or experience. Just as the neurodivergent spectrum of presentation manifests many different "looks," life as a neurodivergent child can look many ways depending on the individual, their strengths, support needs, and the environments they are navigating. As Dr. Stephen Shore has famously coined, "If you have met one child with autism, then you have met one child with autism." This quote could easily say if you have met one neurodivergent child, then you have met one neurodivergent child. While it is essential to acknowledge the individualized nature of being neurodivergent, there are some commonalities for those living neurodivergent lives.

A Systemic Issue: There are a myriad of ways that a neurodivergent person may have support needs. The support provided or lack of support (ableist experiences) will permeate throughout home life, extended family, school environment, community, and job environment. When working with neurodivergent children, it is critical to remember how all-encompassing being neurodivergent is for the person's life.

School Challenges: From the very beginnings of daycare and preschool and throughout college completion, neurodivergent individuals often face an up-hill battle in most educational settings. The school setting can present some of the greatest challenges to a neurodivergent child. The social and communication demands, processing requirements, sensory experiences, behavior judgments, and widely dynamic and changing environments present in every school day can create great dysregulation for neurodivergent children.

Family Navigation: Neurodivergence often affects the whole family, and the whole family affects the neurodivergent child. It is not unusual for the family's time, decisions, and resources to center around the neurodivergent child. The family system can become a place of great support or another dysregulating environment. Family expectations may not align with the neurodiversity paradigm and may need to be addressed.

Therapies: Therapies, programs, and interventions may cover a whole variety of support needs depending on the individual. Therapies can also be time-consuming and expensive. Additionally, there is a long history of therapies focusing on trying to change the neurodivergent child into a neurotypical child and thus creating more mental health needs instead of being helpful.

Self-Acceptance: Neurodivergent individuals are often in a continuous process of trying to understand themselves, their neurodivergent identity, how to navigate the world around them, and how to advocate for the world around them to dissolve barriers and create support. Gaining self-awareness of these issues will be critical for neurodivergent children to live their most regulated and autonomous lives. Understanding the role masking may have played in developing the neurodivergent's personality may create a need for unlearning and accepting who they truly are.

Educating Others: Neurodivergent individuals can find much of their time spent educating others about neurodiversity, specifically how their own neurodivergence manifests and describes them. Although education and awareness initiatives continue to increase, there still exists much inaccurate information, ignorance, and stereotyping regarding neurodivergence. Unfortunately, some neurodivergent individuals have found it easier to not disclose they are neurodivergent because of the mislabeling and stigmatization that can occur. Inevitably, neurodivergent people will find themselves in situations where it will be necessary to educate those around them about neurodiversity and how to be neurodiversity-affirming. Neurodivergents have reported that this is exhausting work and are greatly in need of allies to help with this education.

There are several approaches that advertise working with neurodivergent children. Many of these approaches offer individual and group modalities – DIR/

Floortime, Integrated Play Groups, Applied Behavioral Analysis, Replays, etc. There are multiple protocols and too many to list. These approaches are not created equal regarding being neurodiversity informed and affirming and are not absent of ableist ideas. Many historical approaches do not affirm or provide very little affirming constructs. Some advertised neurodivergent approaches include a focus on play and some type of "social skills" gains, but only play therapy theories focus on the natural therapeutic powers of play, therapeutic relationship development as a change agent, and viewing play as a natural process rather than something to be used to gain compliance.

Play Therapy Groups

Knell (1997) stated that play therapy groups developed in part because patterns of behavior emerged in children in group environments that were not present in the play of individual children. Groups focusing on children have grown in the past decade. Professionals have discovered that processes in groups cannot be replicated in individual work, and the group atmosphere holds much benefit for children. Sweeney et al. (2014) proposed that groups serve as a practice field for the outside world, and the expressive and projective nature of playgroups enable this practice to become real, thus easier to transfer and generalize to other settings and experiences.

Group play therapy is a process of exploration that group members embark upon, and the therapist has the privilege of partnering in. While the therapist may direct the group play therapy process, the underlying premise is that the therapist is a witness to the process, a fellow sojourner with the group members. It is upon this attitude that group members feel safe to explore, both with the therapist and with other group members (Sweeney et al., 2014).

Children learn about themselves and others in therapeutic play groups. This is facilitated because the expressive play process promotes communication. Thus, they learn as they observe and listen to the group play therapist and other group members. This is a phenomenological experience, as they perceive the therapists and other group members' interactions with them. Group members realize that their uniqueness is not just acceptable; it is valued and prized (Sweeney et al., 2014).

The group play therapy experience can hold many benefits for a child. The involvement in group work lends itself to an exploration and growth that cannot always be duplicated in individual therapy experiences. Sweeney and Homeyer (1999) proposed several points for the benefits of employing group play therapy:

1   They provide opportunities for vicarious learning and catharsis.
2   They provide the opportunity for self-growth and self-exploration.
3   They provide opportunities to anchor clients to the world of reality.
4   They provide an opportunity to gain insight into the client's everyday life.

5 They provide the opportunity to "practice" for everyday life within a safe environment.
6 They provide the opportunity for relationship development.

Play therapy groups are therapeutic sessions facilitated by trained play therapy professionals. A group of children engage in various forms of play (from non-directed to directed) to express themselves, explore their emotions, and work through any psychological or social challenges they may be facing. A typically organized play therapy group would consist of the following elements:

Facilitator(s): A trained therapist leads the group sessions. There may be multiple facilitators depending on the size of the group. They create a safe and supportive environment for children to express themselves through play.

Group Composition: Typically, a group would consist of children within a similar age range or dealing with similar issues. Groups may be formed around themes like sensory needs, grief, trauma, or social interaction.

Activities: If the group is more directive, there will likely be interventions or activities involved. The activities can vary widely depending on the goals of the group and the play preferences of the children. These activities may include movement games, board games, art-related activities, video games, etc.

Nondirective Play: If a group has this focus, there would be no activities or interventions introduced by the facilitator. Children would have unstructured time to play with various toys, art supplies, or other materials provided by the therapist. This allows them to express themselves in a non-verbal way or however they want through their play.

Structured Play: If the group has a more directive element, the facilitator will introduce specific interventions, games, exercises, or activities designed to help children explore the topics or goals of the group.

Expressive Creation: In this type of group, the children may engage in drawing, painting, or other art and creative activities to express their feelings, experience sensory awareness, understand regulation, or address whatever the focus goals of the group may be.

Sand Tray Therapy: A specific type of therapeutic approach where children use a tray filled with sand and various miniature objects to create scenes that represent their thoughts and emotions.

Role-Playing: A more directive element where children may act out scenarios to practice something to help with a targeted need area or group goal such as safety awareness or problem-solving.

Storytelling: A more directive element where the facilitator may use bibliotherapy, video stories, or puppets to help children understand and process their experiences.

Expression and Communication: Regardless of the specific process, play therapy focused groups offer children a safe and non-threatening way to express their thoughts and feelings. Through play, children can communicate things that they may struggle to articulate verbally.

Building Relationships: Group play therapy allows children to interact with their peers in a safe and supportive environment. This can help them develop relationships, friendships, and a sense of belonging.

Therapeutic Goals: Goals for children may vary depending on the group theme and purpose. Regardless, the overarching goal of any play therapy group is to improve the overall well-being of the children participating.

Parent Involvement: Depending on the structure and purpose of the group, parents may be involved in some aspects of the play therapy groups. This involvement can include parent training, family therapy sessions, or regular updates from the therapist on the child's progress.

In general, play therapy groups offer children a valuable opportunity to explore their thoughts and feelings, address mental health needs, and build connections with others in a supportive and therapeutic setting. Play therapy groups for neurodivergent children adhere to the basic concepts found in any play therapy group but are tailored to meet the specific needs and affirming understandings of neurodivergent children (autistic, ADHD children, sensory differences, learning differences, etc.). Studies have shown that compared to neurotypical children, neurodivergent children are less involved in group play and social activities, inconsistently initiate play, and respond to peer play requests (Chester et al., 2019). This highlights the need to understand the neurodivergent social, relational, and group experience and the uniqueness of these constructs for neurodivergent people.

Hull (2014) discussed the benefits of groups for neurodivergent children, including connecting children and adolescents and adding another dimension of peer support and connection, providing a place to discover there are others like them, a chance to have a positive peer/social experience, providing encouragement, a sense of safety, a social place that communicates to the child they are valuable and accepted and will not be judged or rejected, and providing children with the message they are not "weird," "wrong," "damaged," or "unlovable." Hull (2014) further outlined specific neurodivergent benefits for children in participating in group work, including understanding and addressing Alexithymia, helping with social navigation needs, perspective-taking, increasing self-worth and self-confidence, and establishing a sense of identity.

The therapist implementing play therapy groups will need to go beyond the basics of understanding group work when working with neurodivergent clients. When facilitating play groups for neurodivergent children, there are some additional and important considerations:

Specialized Facilitation: Trained therapists with expertise in working with neurodivergent children should lead the groups. They should possess an understanding of the unique support needs and strengths associated with being neurodivergent and construct the group experience through a neurodiversity-affirming lens.

Sensory Considerations: Many neurodivergent children have sensory differences. Play therapy groups for neurodivergent children often incorporate sensory-friendly environments, such as providing options for different textures, lighting, sounds, and spaces for both sensory-seeking and sensory-avoidant behaviors.

Structured and Predictable Routines: Many neurodivergent children benefit from clear routines, structure, and a predictable experience. The group therapy sessions should have a structure and follow a predictable format, with consistent rituals or activities to start and end each session, helping to provide a sense of safety and regulation for the child's nervous system.

Visual Supports: Visual aids, such as schedules, picture cards, or social stories, may be used to help neurodivergent children understand the sequence of activities, expectations, and transitions during play therapy sessions. These can also be beneficial in helping children understand when group time is ending.

Choice and Flexibility: While structure is important, allowing for flexibility and accommodating individual needs and preferences is essential. Neurodivergent children may have specific interests, sensory preferences, and ways of communicating and navigating socially that influence their participation in the playgroup. Being flexible with differences and providing choices within the activities and participation level can empower children and communicate value to their neurodivergent identity.

Social Elements: By design, play therapy groups for neurodivergent children will incorporate being around and some level of interaction with peers. This can be a powerful and meaningful experience for a neurodivergent child. It does require a level of caution for the facilitator, as social elements may be anxiety-producing and dysregulating for some neurodivergent children. Each neurodivergent child's way of navigating socially should be respected and valued.

Regulation Needs: Children with neurodivergent conditions may face challenges related to dysregulation and coping with sensory overload or social stressors. Play therapy groups may focus on and provide opportunities for children to practice regulation work in a safe and non-judgmental environment. Even if it is not the focus of the group, the therapist must constantly be mindful of the regulation/dysregulation experience of each of the group members.

Parent/Caregiver Involvement: In many cases, involving parents or caregivers in the group play therapy process is crucial. This involvement may include having parents on standby in an adjacent room if needed to help with a scenario, observing the group sessions, providing additional psychoeducation to parents on how to support their child at home, and actively participating in the group experience with their child.

Play therapy groups for neurodivergent children follow the same basic format as any play therapy group with some necessary considerations for neurodivergence. The aim is to provide a supportive and inclusive environment where children can explore, express themselves, address their needs, and build resilience under the guidance of a neurodiversity-informed and -affirming professional who understands their needs and values their neurodivergent identity.

Doing Better for Neurodivergent Children

Recognizing strengths in neurodivergent children and valuing neurodiversity has significant benefits. It can help children (and their parents) frame their challenges as differences rather than deficits. It can also shed light on instructional approaches that might help to highlight particular strengths. It also normalizes the fact that there are many productive individual members of society who are not neurotypical, and different ways of thinking, processing, and responding can be valuable. When neurotypical individuals understand neurodiversity, neurodivergent children are more accepted and appreciated in the social settings and environments they are navigating.

It is important to focus on the positives when discussing neurodivergent children. Understanding and communicating about a neurodivergent child's strengths and successes is crucial to teaching other children and adults to view neurodivergence through a non-ableist and more positive lens. It is also important to incorporate the neurodivergent child in the conversation, allowing them to express what they feel when they experience sensory challenges, dysregulation, social situations, confusion, etc. Neurodiversity initiatives mean explaining to others that neurodivergent children may process information a little differently and that can change the way they communicate in social situations and how they express themselves when they feel uncomfortable or overwhelmed. Nelly Thomas created the children's picture book *Some Brains: A Book Celebrating Neurodiversity*, which focuses on children discussing neurodivergence. Books such as these can be a valuable tool in helping all people and the child themselves gain better positive awareness about being neurodivergent.

Often, neurodivergent children are seen as having a diagnosis, which usually carries a host of stigmas and negative assumptions about how the child is going to present. This view diminishes and hides any recognition of the child's strengths. It creates a situation that makes the child a behavior (usually negative behavior) instead of a fully functioning, unique individual with a host of abilities and strengths despite their possible needs. Professionals across multiple settings can support neurodivergent children, as many neurodivergent children find themselves on the opposite end of support. Many are criticized, misunderstood, and treated badly by others. As professionals increase their awareness and understanding of neurodivergence, they are positioned to walk alongside neurodivergent children and offer support, encouragement, and validation.

Grant (2023) stated there are multiple ways therapists can provide meaningful support to neurodivergent children. Support begins with becoming educated and learning about neurodiversity, the neurodiversity paradigm, neurodiversity-affirming principles, and the personal lived experiences of neurodivergent people. Supporting neurodivergent children and adolescents also means supporting parents. Support involves avoiding the judgment of parents and instead aiding, asking how help can be provided, offering psychoeducation about neurodiversity, and listening to their needs and struggles. A sincere attempt to help and provide support can make a successful difference for a neurodivergent child. Some additional ways to support neurodivergent children and adolescents include:

- Get to know the neurodivergent child. Develop a relationship with the child.
- Discover what the child likes and enjoys, their interests, and their play preferences.
- Focus on the child's strengths, what they do well, and recognize their accomplishments.
- Avoid focusing on the child's "negative" behavior and make everything about their behavior.
- Maintain an open mind to continue to learn about neurodivergence.
- Remember the neurodivergent child may have a different navigation style from you.
- Remember the neurodivergent child may need specific environmental support.
- Think about keeping the environment sensory and regulation-friendly.
- Allow and encourage neurodivergent children to be their authentic selves.

The world of neurodivergence is a vast and often complex place with many variables, thoughts, and opinions. Neurodivergent individuals must learn to understand themselves and how their unique person maneuvers in the greater world in which they live. Just as the neurodivergent individual is on a journey, those who work with, interact with, educate, serve, and help those who are neurodivergent are also on a journey. Their journey involves increasing their willingness to understand and increase acceptance of neurodivergent individuals. Their process of becoming neurodiversity-informed and -affirming means being caring and kind and making the effort to value differences and see the strengths that the neurodivergent person brings to any setting. For the neurodiversity-affirming therapist, it is not just learning about neurodiversity but applying that knowledge to the real people they encounter each day.

AutPlay Play and Social Groups

AutPlay Therapy play and social groups utilize play to help neurodivergent children improve their overall well-being. AutPlay groups present a neurodiversity-affirming relational-based framework that integrates elements of established play therapy theories and approaches and can easily be combined with additional interventions. Children and parents can participate in AutPlay groups, and specific focus is given to building the therapeutic relationship as well as building upon the child's natural interests. The self of the child is respected, and their uniqueness is valued. Social interaction and navigation are built upon the child's strengths and play preferences and interests. Group processes and interventions are designed to provide meaning for the child. This book outlines the process of implementing AutPlay play and social groups and can be used as a guide for professionals who work with neurodivergent children. It serves as an affirming resource to establish and implement play and social groups for children and adolescents. Additionally, this book provides professionals with an adaptable protocol and tools necessary to create and lead play therapy groups to assist neurodivergent children with a variety of strengths and challenges.

The AutPlay groups protocol describes how to start a group and highlights various group mechanics to follow that help ensure group success. The appendix provides several forms and documents that are used when beginning a group and tracking documents that can help chart each child's successes. These documents also help professionals collect valuable information when deciding on what type of group to implement. Further, several structured play interventions and activities for helping children and adolescents address a variety of needs are presented for professionals to use during group times.

Professionals can modify and adapt groups to fit their specific needs and are also capable of adding to or taking away from the basic concepts presented in this book. AutPlay play and social groups are flexible and adaptable. There are many successful and affirming ways to expose neurodivergent children and adolescents to group work where they can address their mental health needs. Professionals can feel confident using this approach and integrating methods to meet the unique needs of this underserved, diverse group. AutPlay groups assist children and adolescents by providing a supportive and playful structure to learn and grow. Therapists should strive to maintain a balance between the therapeutic powers of playful relationships and neurodiversity-affirming principles. AutPlay groups support the integration of these components to create the most honoring and sustainable approach to group work.

References

Chester, M., Richdale, A. L., & McGillivray, J. (2019). Group-based social skills training with play for children on the autism spectrum. *Journal of Autism and Developmental Disorders, 49*(6), 2231–2242. https://doi.org/10.1007/s10803-019-03892-7

Grant, R. J. (2023). *AutPlay therapy handbook: Integrative family play therapy with neurodivergent children.* Routledge.

Grant, R. J., Barboa, L., Luck, J., & Obrey, E. (2022). *The complete guide to becoming an autism friendly professional: Working with individuals, groups, and organization.* Routledge.

Higashida, N. (2013). *The reason I jump: The inner voice of a thirteen-year-old boy with autism*. Random House.

Hull, K. B. (2014). *Group therapy techniques with children, adolescents, and adults on the autism spectrum: Growth and connection for all ages*. Jason Aronson.

Knell, S. M. (1997). *Cognitive behavioral play therapy*. Rowman & Littlefield.

Koenig, K. (2012). *Practical social skills for autism spectrum disorders*. W. W. Norton.

Panzano, L. (2018). Five research-based strengths associated with autism. *Stages Learning Materials*.https://blog.stageslearning.com/blog/five-research-based-strengths-associated-with-autism.

Sweeney, D. S., Baggerly, J. N., & Ray, D. C. (2014). *Group play therapy: A dynamic approach*. Routledge.

Sweeney, D. S., & Homeyer, L. E. (1999). Group play therapy. In D. S. Sweeney & L. E. Homeyer (Eds.), *The handbook of group play therapy: How to do it, how it works, whom it's best for* (pp. 3–14). Jossey-Bass.

Chapter 1

Neurodiversity

Understanding Neurodiversity

Neurodiversity refers to the idea that neurological differences, such as those seen in autistic and other neurodivergent people, reflect normal variations in brain development. Neurodiversity is often contrasted with the "medical model," which views autism, ADHD, learning differences, sensory differences, and pretty much all neurodivergence as disorders to prevent, treat, or cure. There has been a push (primarily led by the neurodivergent community) to move away from this idea of pathology and more toward awareness and acceptance of the diversity of neurotypes.

Neurodiversity and neurodivergent people have always existed although there has not always been a formal language for identification purposes. The neurodiversity movement has been in existence for the past few decades but has seen significant growth in the last 10–15 years. Several autistic and other neurodivergent people were discussing and conceptualizing the diversity of brains in the 1990s. The word *neurodiversity* saw its first formal publication in 1998 with the work of Judy Singer and Harvey Blume. Singer is an Australian sociologist who used the word to recognize that every human brain develops in a unique way. No two brains are exactly alike; therefore, there's no real "normal" brain (Singer, 2017).

In this aspect, we are all neurodiverse. It is important to recognize, however, that social and cultural norms dictate to a degree what range of neurodiversity is "typical," "expected," or "within the norm." From these concepts, the word *neurodivergent* comes into play. Although all of us are neurodiverse, we are not all neurodivergent. The term neurodivergent would signify those whose brains, therefore their style of thinking, learning, interacting, etc., vary significantly from the mainstream neurotypical created standard. Again, it is important to remember that this norm can vary significantly depending on region and culture. From the words neurodiversity and neurodivergent comes the *neurodiversity movement*, a movement to support neurodivergents and help them feel accepted, included, and appreciated in society. This movement can be seen as a social, political, and human rights platform.

DOI: 10.4324/9781003468370-2

Robison (2013) proposed that many individuals who embrace the concept of neurodiversity believe that people with differences do not need to be cured; they need help and accommodation instead. They look at the pool of diverse humanity and see – in the middle – the range of different thinking that's made humanity's progress in science and the creative arts possible. When 99 neurologically identical people fail to solve a problem, it's often the 1% fellow who's different who holds the key. Yet that person may be disabled or disadvantaged most or all of the time. To neurodiversity proponents, people are disabled because they are at the edges of the bell curve, not because they are sick or broken.

Robison (2013) furthered that to many neurodiversity proponents, talk of "cure" feels like an attack on their very being. They detest those words for the same reason other groups detest talk of "curing gayness" or "passing for white," and they perceive the accommodation of neurological differences as a similarly charged civil rights issue. If their diversity is part of their makeup, they believe it's their right to be accepted and supported "as is." They should not be made into something else – especially against their will – to fit some imagined societal ideal.

To better understand neurodiversity requires an understanding of cultural humility. Cultural humility is a process of self-reflection and discovery in order to build honest and trustworthy relationships. Cultural humility is a lifelong process of self-reflection and self-critique whereby the individual not only learns about another's culture, but one starts with an examination of their own beliefs and cultural identities (Tervalon & Murray-Garcia, 1998). This critical consciousness is more than just self-awareness. It requires a person to reflect and analyze to understand their own assumptions, biases, and values (Kumagai & Lypson, 2009). Individuals must look at their own background and social environment and how it has shaped their experience. Cultural humility cannot be obtained through a class or book reading. It is viewed as an ongoing, lifelong process.

Yeager & Bauer-Wu (2013) proposed that cultural humility does not focus on competence or confidence and recognizes that the more you are exposed to cultures different from your own, you often realize how much you don't know about others. That is where humility comes in. Humility requires courage and flexibility. Ideas of ableism, where the underlying idea implies that the problem is due to the difference, are abandoned. The strengths and challenges of individuals and groups are explored as well as the advantages and privileges of certain group memberships.

The Hogg Staff (2019) proposed three things that should be understood for cultural humility. These points have been adapted with an understanding and example toward neurodiversity:

1 *We Move between Several Different Cultures*: Though the term "culture" is often used when describing different ethnic or religious affiliations, most people experience and participate in different cultures just by moving through

their daily lives. For example, a person's family or home culture will likely have distinctly different qualities and behavioral expectations than their work culture, school culture, or social group culture. Neurodivergence is viewed as an identity and thus a culture. As such, the constructs that manifest in cultural humility work include neurodiversity as much as any other type of diversity. Because the overall purpose of practicing cultural humility is to be aware of one's own values and beliefs, it is important to understand that those notions come from the combination of cultures that people experience in their everyday lives. A person cannot begin to understand the makeup and context of another person's life without being aware and reflective of their own background and situation first.

Many individuals will know someone who is neurodivergent – a friend, a family member, or a colleague. Some people may be neurodivergent them-selves and do not realize it. It is highly likely that everyone will encounter a neurodivergent person in their day-to-day lives. What do you think about neurodiversity? How does it manifest in terms of what you have been taught about disabled people? Understanding where you are at and where you have come from becomes vitally important in recognizing your own ableist ideas and working to provide affirming support.

2 *Cultural Humility Is Distinct from Cultural Competency*: It is important to know the differences between cultural humility and closely related concepts like cultural competency. Cultural competency is a tool for being aware of other cultures and people groups different from your own and the major-ity society. The shortcomings of this practice, however, have been identified by researchers who reviewed frequently used cultural competency measures. They found that in many frequently used competency measures, the majority societal presentation was viewed as the norm, such as whiteness with race and neurotypical with neurotype. Cultural incompetence is then framed as be-ing due to a lack of knowledge about marginalized groups. In short, the goal of cultural competency is to learn about the other person's culture rather than reflect on one's own background. Cultural competency serves as a beginning but does not fully provide what is needed for marginalized people groups to experience full inclusion and acceptance. It falls short of the lifelong process of self-reflection that is synonymous with cultural humility.

Cultural competence can best be understood in neurodivergence by the popularized autism awareness day and month. The focus of this campaign is to help those who are not autistic (neurotypical people) be more aware that autistic people exist. The deeper premise of the awareness campaign im-plies that autistic people struggle, and you need to be aware and care about them, essentially have pity on them. This manifests a great deal of ableist thought. While awareness of autism and neurodivergent people is a basic good thought, it is an appreciation that eliminates ableist ideas and places the neurodivergent person in an equity position. Cultural humility calls for a person to not just be aware of others but examine their own bias and grow in an appreciation for diversity. In this case, neurodiversity.

3 *Cultural Humility Requires Historical Awareness*: It is not enough to think about one's own values, beliefs, and social position within the context of the present moment. In order to practice true cultural humility, a person must also be aware of and sensitive to historic realities like legacies of violence and oppression against certain groups of people. For example, the historic institutionalization and dignity removal of autistic and other neurodivergent people, especially those with high support needs. The ableist beliefs that created systems where neurodivergent people were viewed as less than a "normal" human and either needed stringent "treatment" to make them "normal" or placed away someone out of site. In order to build trust, the historic, systemic reasons for mistrust must be excavated and made visible. By recognizing the failures of the past, researchers, clinicians, providers, and advocates can all contribute to building a better future that is founded in practices of cultural humility.

Working with neurodivergent children and offering groups to help address their mental health needs sounds like a useful endeavor. For the most part, if executed through an affirming process, they certainly can be useful. Any efforts toward neurodivergent children (including mental health group work) must begin with an understanding of a person's own ableist ideas and conditioning. Further, the professional should commit to an ongoing cultural humility process regarding neurodiversity. This chapter will focus on key terminology and constructs important for professionals to be aware of so they can understand the neurodivergent experience, implement neurodiversity-affirming constructs, and best meet the needs of their neurodivergent clients. Examples of these terms will be given as well to provide further clarification and understanding. Special emphasis will be placed on mental health professionals, especially those who provide play therapy. These professionals need to understand the terms to be advocates for their neurodivergent clients. It is important to understand that some of these terms may be unknown to the reader, and that is acceptable.

The field of neurodiversity-affirming care changes often and can be difficult to navigate. All professionals are life-long learners, and it's helpful to understand this and be receptive toward new learning and growth. Readers may also feel uncomfortable or defensive with some of the examples that are given in this chapter. There is a real possibility that an ableist statement, for example, may be one that the reader felt was acceptable. It may also be a statement that the reader has communicated or continues to communicate. Therapy professionals are often hard on themselves and can feel guilt and shame even when unaware of some new practices. As the reader navigates this chapter, it may be helpful to expect learning new terms and examples of which they are unaware. From this point, the professional can then assess within how they feel about neurodiversity concepts and then develop a plan of action in their working with clients. It is through humility and receptiveness to growth that we can become an important part of the neurodiversity movement.

Key Terminology, Constructs, and Examples

Neurodiversity: As described earlier in this chapter, all humans are neurodiverse. Neurodiversity is the understanding that all humans are unique and have individualized differences. These diversities can also follow an individual's race, ethnicity, gender, sexual orientation, status, age, etc.

• Examples: Learning examples could include how some individuals are visual learners, while others are auditory learners. Social examples include the range of extroversion versus introversion. How individuals express themselves also shows their individual neurodiversity, with some expressing through words, others through visual examples or through movement, such as sign language. Everyone has a neurodiversity profile of sorts, which explains how they best learn, understand, socialize, express, and more.

Neurodivergent: Individuals are considered neurodivergent when their minds function in ways that diverge significantly from the dominant societal norm of "normal." There are specific diagnoses that are classified as neurodivergent, but a diagnosis is not required to be neurodivergent.

• Examples: autism, ADHD, learning differences, sensory differences, giftedness, highly sensitive children, intellectual developmental disorder, developmental disabilities, etc. are examples of diagnoses that fall within the neurodivergent spectrum. These diagnoses may have individuals experience social, learning, expression, movement, and sensory profiles that vary significantly from the social norm. This "social norm" is heavily dependent upon social and cultural norms within each society; for example, functions that may be considered neurodivergent in North America may not be seen as neurodivergent in Asia.

Neuro Minority: Any group, such as autistics, who differ from the majority population in terms of brain function and social, emotional, and behavioral traits. Under the umbrella of neurodivergent, there are multiple neurominorities. These minorities may have distinct presentations.

• Examples: The diagnoses of autism, ADHD, learning differences, Tourette syndrome, sensory differences, etc. are each neurominority group, but all are neurodivergent.

Neurodiversity Paradigm: This is a specific perspective on neurodiversity. It is an approach in which neurodiversity is viewed as being not only natural but valuable. It dismisses the idea that there exists a "normal" brain or a "right" way of functioning. It recognizes the effect that a society's rules and norms can have on misunderstanding those who do not fall into these norms.

- Examples: Professionals who follow this approach will welcome all clients, regardless of diagnosis or ability. They will be open to learning about each client's unique self through listening both to the client and the significant people in the client's life. Professionals will work on therapy planning based on the client's needs and desires. They will find ways to make interventions fun for the client and relatable. These professionals must be open, flexible, and willing to learn while strongly believing that the client knows themselves and their needs best.

Neurodiversity Movement: The neurodiversity movement is a social justice movement. This movement seeks the rights and respect of all neurodivergents. The expectation is that all neurodivergents are fully integrated into society and accepted for who they are.

- Examples: Professionals who are part of the neurodiversity movement will find themselves advocating for their neurodivergent clients often. They will guide the clients' parents into a better understanding of their neurodivergent child. They will consult with school personnel to ensure that the neurodivergent client's educational needs are being met. They may need to reach out into their community to educate others on the neurodiversity paradigm. Most importantly, these professionals will continue to check themselves to ensure they are operating in a neurodiversity-friendly manner.

Ableism: Grant (2023) described ableism as the discrimination, oppression, and social prejudice against people with disabilities based on the belief that typical abilities are superior. At its heart, ableism is rooted in the assumption that disabled people require "fixing" and devalues people based on real or perceived disability. Hayden-Laurelut et al. (2013) furthered that ableism has been defined as a network of beliefs, processes, and practices that produces a particular kind of self that is projected as the perfect, species-typical, and therefore essential and fully human. Disability is then cast as a diminished state of being human.

Like racism and sexism, ableism classifies entire groups of people as "less than" and includes harmful stereotypes, misconceptions, and generalizations of people with disabilities. Ableism can take an intentional presentation. Individuals can be purposely discriminatory or devaluing of those with disabilities, including neurodivergent individuals.

They may say or do things because they believe or feel that the disabled are not as worthy, important, or valuable as nondisabled or neurotypical individuals. Most of the intentional and direct occurrences come in the form of microaggressions – commonplace daily verbal, behavioral, or environmental slights – that communicate hostile, derogatory, or negative attitudes toward stigmatized or culturally marginalized groups. Many acts of ableism likely happen unintentionally and indirectly. Individuals often unknowingly commit microaggressions or support processes or systems that are ableist. Many systems that are currently in place and taught to or experienced by individuals as they grow are laden with ableist ideas and practices.

Many people grow up in these systems and are conditioned in ableist ways of thinking and being without being aware. All people have a responsibility to challenge their own beliefs and actions as well as the systems they navigate to eradicate ableist ideas.

Reeve (2000) identified ableism in counseling practice, where counselors employ a predominantly medical model of disability that risks discounting alternative relational understandings. In counseling/therapy, disability is constructed in relation to the normal. Disability is always understood as a problematic deviation from the normal, as an imperfection when judged against what is considered normative. There is a risk of needing to "fix" or "cure" something that is actually a part of or who the person identifies as. This can manifest through the therapist's attitude, approach, and microaggressions in interventions and treatment goals. It is important that therapists understand the harm that has been done historically to neurodivergent children. Understanding the problematic past can help prevent this type of treatment from happening in the present and future.

• Examples: Addressing ableism is a sensitive topic and can cause professionals to feel defensive. This is an area in which we are constantly learning new information and are expected to change as we learn. All of us have a lot to learn when it comes to our own ableist ideas. It is important for us to "sit with" any defensiveness that comes up as we are learning ways to improve our thoughts, words, and actions. There are some forms of ableism that are obvious to many professionals. These would include expecting an autistic to display eye contact, telling an ADHD'er that their way of communicating is wrong, or insisting that someone with a math disability is not allowed to use a manipulative to learn a particular concept. There are also subtle forms of ableism that professionals may not be aware of. Examples of subtle ableism include stating an autistic is "high functioning" or "low functioning," believing that an ADHD'er could focus better on homework if they have excellent focus playing a video game, or believing that someone who is intellectually disabled will not be able to live alone or have a romantic relationship. There is also a possibility that professionals will encounter clients who have internalized ableist thoughts about themselves. They may have an adult client believe that they are lazy despite having ADHD or that they are being difficult with clothing choices despite having sensory differences. Professionals will need to work gently with these clients to help them unmask and learn new ideas that better fit with self-advocation. Professionals can best work on their own ableist thoughts and ideas by keeping current with knowledge in the neurodiversity community, especially from those who themselves are neurodivergent. They must be accepting of others "calling them out" if they do indeed make an ableist statement. Finally, professionals can seek additional training and consultation with other professionals to help dig deep within themselves to become more neurodiversity-affirming. It is important to remember that this is a lifelong process; we never stop learning.

Neurodiversity-Affirming: A set of processes based on a neurodiversity-informed lens. The action of learning about the neurodiversity movement, the neurodiversity paradigm, ableism, etc. to be affirming to neurodivergent clients.

- Examples: Professionals who wish to be neurodiversity-affirming need to do a lot of work. They will need to stay aware of the growing research in the field of neurodiversity. This can be done through attending trainings, readings, research reviews, and more. As important as it is for professionals to do academic work, it is equally important for them to be doing the "self work." Professionals must continually look within themselves to explore any ableist or non-affirming thoughts they may hold. They must sit with these thoughts and allow any defensiveness to arise. Professionals need to question their defensiveness and seek out consultation or supervision if they notice it is not alleviating. Often, good self-care can help with this affirming work. As professionals become used to this difficult work, they often become less defensive as they learn more about how they can improve to be advocates for their clients. It is especially important for professionals to remember that this work is never complete; it is a lifelong journey to learn more, and then discover within how this learning is being understood.

Medical Model: Pertaining to neurodivergence, the medical model is how various diagnoses that are on the neurodivergence spectrum are defined. This model uses the DSM as its diagnostic tool and is the primary method for diagnosis.

- Examples: Professionals need to be aware that they will often receive assessment information from their client's diagnosis team. This information is based on the medical model and may include, as one example, the "level" of autism their client fits into (Level 1, 2, or 3). Language used in these assessments is often viewed as negative and filled with potentially ableist language. Examples of troublesome words include deficits, disabled, unable, social skills, high functioning, low functioning, etc. Often the diagnosis team may suggest therapies that are seen as ableist within the neurodivergent community. It is very important that professionals act as advocates for their clients when receiving this information. Professionals may need to inform parents that, while this diagnostic information is important for assessment, it is based on the medical model of diagnosis, which can be ableist and non-affirming. We can work with parents in showing them ways to adjust this information into language that is affirming. We can also work with the clients to better understand what this diagnosis means to them in an affirming manner, for example, by focusing on the many things the child can do rather than what they can't do.

Social Model of Disability: The social model of disability has been created as a response to the medical model of disability. The social model of disability believes that individuals are not disabled by their diagnosis or condition. Rather, it is a society that creates this disability by its' attitudes and beliefs. This model believes that society tends to be an ableist majority that can greatly affect the needs, behaviors, and actions of neurodivergent.

Olkin (2022) stated that in the social model, disability is seen as one aspect of a person's identity, much like race/ethnicity, gender, etc. From this perspective, disability is believed to result from a mismatch between the disabled person and the environment (both physical and social). It is this environment that creates the handicaps and barriers, not the disability. From this perspective, the way to address disability is to change the environment and society, rather than people with disabilities. Negative stereotypes, discrimination, and oppression serve as barriers to environmental change and full inclusion.

Buder and Perry (2022) proposed that the social model of disability suggests that if societies were set up and constructed in a way that was accessible for people with disabilities, those individuals would not be restricted from full participation in the world around them. In other words, the social model of disability views the origins of disability as the mental attitudes and physical structures of society, rather than a medical condition faced by an individual. Essentially, the social model says that individual limitations are not the cause of disability. Rather, it is society's failure to provide appropriate services and adequately ensure that the needs of disabled people are taken into account in societal organizations. Simply constructing sidewalks and entrances that are wheelchair accessible, for example, can turn a disability into an ability.

- Examples: A classic example of this could be the use of eye contact. In Western society, maintaining eye contact was viewed as a sign of focus, attention, and respect. When some neurodivergents did not maintain eye contact, the medical model of disability viewed this as a problem that needed to be fixed. Many therapy protocols would focus on a treatment plan goal of their clients maintaining eye contact. The social model of disability would posit that not maintaining eye contact is not an issue or a problem and that individuals can hold focus and attention without showing eye contact. It is instead the ableist view of society that maintaining eye contact is important that has created this to be an issue.

Neurotypical (neuronormative): Individuals are considered neurotypical when their minds function in ways that do not diverge significantly from the dominant societal norm of "normal." Neurotypical individuals are within the societal range of "acceptable" behavior.

• Examples: Neurotypical individuals are those who have found it rather easy to move about in the world. They typically can understand and function with social, emotional, mental, communication, and other societal norms. It may be second nature for these individuals to navigate through the world, that they may be unaware of the great difficulties it causes for others. This does not mean that neurotypical individuals do not have their own challenges, and many diagnoses are not considered neurodivergent. But, overall, neurotypical individuals are within the norm of societal acceptance.

Stimming: Stimming is the repetitive movement, action, vocalization, etc. in order to self-regulate. It is seen to be a coping mechanism to help with relaxation, calming, regulation, and feelings expression. It can be seen in the neurodivergent population, although neurotypicals may stim as well.

• Examples: Examples of stimming include body rocking, swaying, bouncing, blinking, hand flapping, pacing, humming, vocalizations, or thoughts. In the past, some therapeutic protocols called for the reduction and extinction of stimming behavior. Professionals have since learned that stimming is natural and often an effective way to help with emotion regulation. Professionals who work with clients who stim should normalize this action and advocate for them when necessary. If the stim is causing harm to the client or others, the professional can help discover a replacement stim.

Echolalia: The repetition of words, often words just spoken by another person. Echolalia is seen as automatic, non-voluntary behavior and a type of stimming.

• Examples: Examples of echolalia may be individuals who immediately repeat the speech of another or repeat the speech of another after a period of time. It may be repeated in the exact same cadence and/or tone. It may be repeated multiple times in multiple settings. At one time, echolalia was considered "meaningless speech" and treatment plan goals may involve eliminating echolalia. It is now seen as a possible factor due to the differences in language development within individuals and a possible stimming action. Echolalia does not need to be corrected or worked on and is an acceptable form of communication and regulation.

Receptive Language: This is the ability of individuals to understand and comprehend spoken language.

- Examples: Receptive language is different from expressive language in that it involves the understanding and comprehension of spoken language either heard or read. Expressive language, in comparison, is the ability to communicate through verbal or non-verbal means. Many neurodivergents can communicate exceptionally well, especially over topics that interest them. However, being able to process, understand, and comprehend what others are communicating to them may be more difficult. Often, professionals may assume that their clients have advanced receptive language abilities due to their client's advanced verbal language skills, but this may be a faulty assumption. Individuals can have advanced verbal language skills while having challenging receptive language abilities. It is important for professionals to understand the differences between expressive and receptive language and advocate for their clients by ensuring that others in their lives understand this as well.

Alexithymia: This is described as individuals who have great difficulty in recognizing, labeling, and expressing their own emotions in traditional ways. Lo (2021) stated psychological construct is used to describe people who struggle with feeling and expressing emotions. It represents a reduced ability, or sometimes a complete inability, to be connected with the internal emotive signals your body sends you. If a person has alexithymia, they do not only have trouble knowing how they feel, but they may also struggle to tell how others feel. This can make a person socially anxious as they cannot read non-verbal cues. They may come across as socially awkward or lacking in humor.

- Examples: It is important for professionals to know that alexithymia exists in approximately 10% of the population and more often in the neurodivergent population. It can be helpful to remember that this may be a cause as to why some clients may be unable to come up with words to adequately express how they are feeling. Particular care needs to be given to clients with alexithymia to affirm their needs for understanding and not assume that they are unfeeling or uncaring.

Dysregulation: Dysregulation occurs in everyone and is an expected part of life. Dysregulation can exist at different levels within a person. This is sometimes referred to as the window of tolerance model. When a person's system has become too overwhelmed, we see the classic dysregulation meltdown. This is an out-of-control state where the person is greatly struggling. Typically for neurodivergent children, there is something or more than one thing that is causing their system to become dysregulated. Part of addressing dysregulation is understating what is dysregulating the child and making appropriate changes to environments or implementing supports.

- Examples: Neurodivergent clients often have difficulties with coping with dysregulation. The professional can first work with the client on normalizing dysregulation and making sure they understand that dysregulation happens to everyone, every day. Regulation thermometers, scaling emotions, and learning feeling intensity vocabulary can all help clients manage the normalization of being dysregulated. Some neurodivergent clients may have a smaller window of tolerance and hyper/hypo arouse more quickly. In these cases, it is helpful for the professional to work with the client on coping tools that can help with this uncomfortable feeling. As always, the neurodiversity-affirming professional will choose coping skills based on the client's interests and likes.

Masking: Neurodivergent masking, camouflaging, or compensating is a conscious or unconscious suppression of natural neurodivergent responses. It is hiding or controlling behaviors, interactions, and natural ways of being that may be viewed as inappropriate in situations. This occurs when individuals hide their natural selves to conform to the social norm of behavior. Reasons for this include avoiding rejection, sustaining a job, and being accepted. Neurodivergent children may feel the need to present or perform social behaviors that are considered neurotypical or may hide their preferred behaviors in order to be accepted and fit in.

A neurodivergent child may mask to avoid being outed or harassed at school or other social settings. It can help a person feel safe from misunderstandings or aggression, but this act of self-preservation takes a toll on self-esteem and self-identity. Some neurodivergent individuals report unintentional masking in which they were not aware they were masking. Others report having masked for so long that they have difficulty knowing who they really are. Masking can contribute to burnout, which occurs when the challenge of life exceeds a child's resources. It can lead to serious health physical and mental health problems; research outcomes show that masking often leads to depression, anxiety, and poor self-worth.

Bennie (2022) outlined common signs of masking, why neurodivergent individuals would mask, and the negative effects of masking.

Signs of Masking

Forcing or faking eye contact during conversations, imitating smiles and other facial expressions mimicking gestures, hiding or minimizing personal interests, developing a repertoire of rehearsed responses to questions, scripting conversations, pushing through intense sensory discomfort including loud noises, and disguising stimming behaviors (hiding a jiggling foot or trading a preferred movement for one that's less obvious).

Why Does Someone Mask?

Wanting to blend in and not stand out from the crowd, to obtain a job, meet the job qualifications, or improve employment opportunities, concerns about personal safety and well-being (bullying, verbal or emotional attacks, assault, and intimidation), to increase connections and relationships with others, to lessen the risk of failure in social situations by using structured techniques, thereby reducing uncertainty and increasing confidence in the ability to socialize and to avoid discrimination and negative responses from others.

Negative Effects of Masking

Exhaustion and fatigue, change in self-perception or self-identity (not feeling like one's true self, feeling like a "fake"), increased stress and anxiety, depression, neurodivergent-burnout, a delayed, neurodivergent-related diagnosis, and increased risk of experiencing thwarted belongingness and lifetime suicidality

- Examples: Examples of masking can include acting interested in an activity in which they really aren't, speaking a particular way to be accepted, acting happy when they are scared, suppressing stims, maintaining eye contact, moving a particular way, etc. Professionals can work with clients to improve their self-image as well as find friends who accept them for their true selves. Professionals will need to educate the family of their client to help them see the difficulties chronic masking can have on their child. When working with neurodivergent adults who have masked for years, the professional may notice grief work needing to be done. There can be a sense of "who am I?" with adult clients, and sorrow attached to that question. A great deal of sensitivity is needed when working with neurodivergent adults.

Double Empathy Problem (Theory): This may occur when neurodivergents and neurotypicals are attempting to communicate and have a relationship with each other. Both sides may have difficulties understanding the other, which can cause challenges in the relationships. It highlights the idea that communicating and relationship building are two-way streets; both parties must be sensitive to the other and work together to help the relationship.

ZamZow (2021) proposed that the basis of the theory is that a mismatch between two people can lead to faulty communication. This disconnect can occur at many levels, from conversation styles to how people see the world. The greater the disconnect, the more difficulty the two people will have interacting. In the case of neurodivergence, a communication gap between neurodivergent people and neurotypical people may occur not only because neurodivergent people have trouble understanding neurotypical people but also because neurotypical people have trouble understanding them. The problem, the theory posits, is mutual.

- Examples: In the past, all the impetus to change was placed on the neuro-divergent person. They were taught the "correct" way to express, respond, understand, etc. It is extremely important for professionals to understand the double empathy concept and explain it to their neurodivergent clients as well as the family members of the client. Every person in the relationship has a responsibility to enhance the relationship and must work together to foster a healthy relationship.

Monotropism: When individuals are highly focused on few interests at a time. Such focus is placed on these interests that other things may not be noticed or preferred.

- Examples: In the past, terms such as "rigid thinkers," "perserverators," and others were used to describe neurodivergents who had focused interests. These words are not fully accurate and may suggest that having focused interests is a nega-tive thing. As professionals, we want to encourage our neurodivergent clients to express to us their interests, and we are willing to learn, play, and further under-stand what these interests mean to them. Some neurodivergent clients will want guidance on how to focus on necessary items in which they have no interest. An example of this is homework. When the individual must do their homework to pass school but is completely uninterested in the homework, intervention is often needed. When the client wishes for this, it can be helpful to work with the client on strategies to sustain focus on these disinterested but needed items. One effective strategy is finding ways to "inject" interest in non-preferred activities. For example, a child who loves Minecraft but dislikes math calculations may be more interested in these calculations if taught through a Minecraft lens.

Rejection Sensitive Dysphoria: We all have a reaction to real or perceived rejections. For some of us, this reaction is either mild or short-lasting. Those with rejection-sensitive dysphoria feel an extreme emotional reaction to real or per-ceived rejections. They describe feelings of shame, humiliation, and despair at both intense levels and for long durations. Some share that they exert great effort at getting others to like them to avoid rejections, at a cost to their own true identities.

- Examples: Professionals will want to work gently with their neurodivergent clients who experience rejection-sensitive dysphoria. They will advocate for their clients and inform others that words such as "over sensitive" and "reactive" can be unhelpful. They will normalize the impossibility of having everyone like them. It can be helpful to give examples of famous people who often must rise above a great deal of rejection yet are still navigating the world. Additional work can focus on the "are you sure?" concept to discuss perceived rejections. There are times where perceived rejections can be from many other causes having nothing to do with the client. Finally, mindfulness and sensory strategies can help the client when rejection sensitivity is causing high levels of emotion dysregulation.

Sensory Processing Differences: This is a condition in which the brain has difficulty receiving and responding to sensory information. Sensory information can be overstimulating, neutral, or understimulating. Individuals can feel both oversensitive and undersensitive to various stimuli in their environment. It is important to note that in addition to the five senses, there are additional senses of proprioception, vestibular, and interoception, which can cause needs with neurodivergent clients. Proprioception is the sense that gives us information about movement and the positions of our bodies. It helps with movement and force exerted. Vestibular is the sense that helps us determine where we are in relation to space and helps with balance and coordination. Interoception is the sense that helps us understand our inner selves, such as temperature, hunger, tiredness, and the need to urinate.

* Examples: Professionals should spend time with their clients helping them understand their sensory profile. It can be very dysregulating for clients to feel over and/or understimulated by their sensory input. This dysregulation can result in behaviors that can cause difficulties for our clients. Clients who understand their sensory profiles can learn strategies to avoid or attract certain sensory inputs. Professionals can advocate for their clients having sensory items available for them to use at any time.

This is a sampling of some of the important terminology and constructs to learn when professionals work with the neurodivergent population. This list is not exhaustive, and new terms can be developed at any time. Any one or multiple of these constructs could be present in and affect the AutPlay group process at any time. It is essential that professionals working with neurodivergent clients understand the manifestations and possibilities of what the neurodivergent client may be experiencing. Group goals may even involve addressing one or more of these concepts.

The key for the therapist is to remember that being an advocate for neurodivergent children is a lifelong process of learning and growing. When we know something is more beneficial for neurodivergents, we do it. When we learn a new concept to better help neurodivergents, we learn more and implement it. If we begin to feel defensive or judgmental about a neurodivergent idea, we sit with these feelings and explore why we may be experiencing this judgment. We seek supervision or consultation if needed and continue to learn, not only about the idea but our possible reasons for feeling the judgment. It is only through an honest and thorough introspection of ourselves as professionals that we can ensure our goal of being neurodiversity-affirming.

References

Bennie, M. (2022, January 11). What is autistic masking? *Autism Awareness Centre Inc.* https://autismawarenesscentre.com/what-is-autistic-masking/

Grant, R. J. (2023). *The AutPlay therapy handbook: Integrative family play therapy with neurodivergent children.* Routledge.

Haydon-Laurelut, M., Nunkoosing, K., & Wilcox, E. (2013). Family therapy and dis/ableism: Constructions of disability in family therapy literature. *Human Systems Journal, 24,* 150–162.

Hogg Staff. (2019, November 5). Thress things to know: Cultural humility. *Hogg Foundation for Mental Health.* https://hogg.utexas.edu/3-things-to-know-cultural-humility

Kumagai, A. K., & Lypson, M. L. (2009). Beyond cultural competence: Critical consciousness, social justice, and multicultural education. *Academic Medicine, 84*(6), 782–787.

Lo, I. (2021). Alexithymia: Do you know what you feel? *Psychology Today.* https://www.psychologytoday.com/us/blog/living-emotional-intensity/202102/alexithymia-do-you-know-what-you-feel

Olkin, R. (2022, March 29). Conceptualizing disability: Three models of disability. https://www.apa.org/ed/precollege/psychology-teacher-network/introductory-psychology/disability-models

Reeve, D. (2000). Oppression within the counselling room. *Disability & Society, 15,* 669–682.

Robison, J. E. (2013). What Is Neurodiversity: Neurodiversity means many things to people. *Psychology Today.* https://www.psychologytoday.com/us/blog/my-life-aspergers/201310/what-is-neurodiversity

Singer, J. (2017). *Neurodiversity: The birth of an idea.* Judy Singer (September 5, 2017).

Tervalon, M., & Murray-Garcia, J. (1998). Cultural humility versus cultural competence: A critical distinction in defining physician training outcomes in multicultural education. *Journal of Health Care for the Poor and Underserved, 9*(2), 117–125.

Yeager, K. A., & Bauer-Wu, S. (2013). Cultural humility: Essential foundation for clinical researchers. *Applied Nursing Research, 26*(4), 251–256. https://doi.org/10.1016/j.apnr.2013.06.008

ZamZow, R. (2021). Double empathy, explained. *Spectrum News.* https://www.spectrumnews.org/news/double-empathy-explained/

Chapter 2

Neurodivergent Children and Adolescents

Understanding Neurodivergent Children and Adolescents

Before we present information in this chapter about neurodivergent children, it is important to begin with understating that neurodivergent children are children. Neurodivergent children have a type of diversity that requires understanding, but the professionals working with these children should always understand that they are whole children, not a lesser version or a version that is broken. They are children with a diverse presentation just like any other diverse child (race, gender, religion). With this understanding in mind, there are some important things to understand about neurodivergent children, and this chapter will attempt to cover some of those understandings.

Neurodivergent is a term used to describe individuals whose brains process, learn, or behave differently from what is considered typical neurological development (neurotypical). Generally, neurotypical individuals move through life without having to wonder if their brains are functioning in a standard way. Being neurodivergent has both strengths and sometimes needs. Of the world's population, 15–20% exhibit some form of neurodivergence. It is believed that there are a variety of ways for the brain to work, and the differences of each mind are embraced instead of being viewed as inadequacies. Neurodiversity recognizes that both brain function and behavioral traits are indicators of how varied humans are (The Children's Guide, 2023).

Neurodivergent children may and often do present differently from the neuronormative standard, but different is not wrong. Neurodivergent children may process information uniquely, displaying strengths in certain areas and challenges in others. They may exhibit enhanced or specialized intellectual abilities, allowing them to excel in specific areas. Some neurodivergent children have heightened sensory perception or attention to detail. They may notice subtle patterns, textures, or sounds that others might overlook. Neurodivergent children may exhibit intense focus and attention toward their areas of interest. They can become deeply immersed in specific tasks or subjects, displaying a remarkable

DOI: 10.4324/9781003468370-3

ability to concentrate for extended periods of time. Neurodivergent minds may experience emotional regulation challenges, including a struggle to express their emotions effectively. As a result, they might exhibit heightened emotional responses (The Children's Guide, 2023).

When professionals, families, and communities embrace neurodiversity, it's good for neurodivergent children's mental health, wellbeing, sense of self, and identity. Embracing neurodiversity and being neurodiversity-affirming takes away the pressure for neurodivergent children to behave in neurotypical ways, hide behavior like stimming, mask or hide who they are, or cope with sensory overstimulation. This kind of pressure can be physically and mentally exhausting (raisingchildren.net.au, 2022).

Embracing neurodiversity is also good for society. Neurodivergent people bring many strengths to society. These include strengths in creative, innovative, and analytical thinking and expertise in areas of special interest. Embracing neurodiversity is about accepting, including, celebrating, and supporting neurodivergent children. Their differences are part of natural variation and don't need to be treated or changed. Raisingchildren.net.au (2022) identified several ways to embrace neurodiversity and support neurodivergent children:

1 Acknowledge that neurodivergent children might do things differently from neurotypical children, and doing things differently is okay.
2 Adjust tasks and activities so that neurodivergent children can fully participate.
3 Recognize and make the most of neurodivergent children's skills, especially the skills they're proud of. This may manifest in their play interests and preferences.
4 Help neurodivergent children develop ways of managing everyday tasks and activities that feel natural to them.
5 Do not expect neurodivergent children to change behavior like stimming, which doesn't interfere with their everyday activities.
6 Make sure that schools, sports clubs, social groups, and community organizations include and support neurodivergent children.
7 Talk with children about neurodiversity, neurodivergence, and acceptance. For example, you could say, "Some people's brains work differently from other people."
8 Look for appropriate ways for your child to communicate with neurodivergent friends.
9 Be aware of the language you use. For example, "Do you prefer 'autistic child' or 'child with autism'?"
10 Challenge unhelpful attitudes. For example, you could advocate if your child client is getting bullied at school.
11 Avoid assumptions. For example, there could be many reasons why a child is eating only packaged snacks at a picnic or wearing headphones at the supermarket.

12 Look for ways to make your community more inclusive. For example, you could be part of a petition encouraging the local supermarket to opt into one "quiet hour" a week, when lights are dimmed and no music is played.
13 Talk respectfully about neurodiversity and neurodivergence. You probably know people who are neurodivergent, even if they haven't told you.
14 Make changes to the environment for children with sensory differences or high levels of anxiety; for example, perhaps your office uses quiet spaces, adjusts lighting, or allows children to use sensory items like squishy balls during sessions.
15 Recognize and use play approaches and interventions that suit the diverse learning styles or needs of your child clients.
16 Provide support and education for all children to include neurodivergent children in interactions and play.

There is a considerable history of not supporting, devaluing, and misunderstanding neurodivergent children. It has taken neurodivergent adults through the neurodiversity movement to begin important changes needed to better help our neurodivergent clients. It is important for today's professionals to realize the harm and possible trauma previous therapeutic approaches have caused neurodivergent individuals. We must do better while also understanding the importance of trust between clients and professionals. Past treatment of neurodivergent clients primarily involved a strict, behavioral approach. The neurotypical norm was the basis upon which treatment plan goals were set. There was little to no acceptance of common neurodivergent behaviors. The primary objective was to "fix" the neurodivergent child, meaning they would be or at least look neurotypical.

The focus of treatment planning goals through a neurotypical lens included some of the following increased eye contact, reduction and elimination of stimming behaviors, how to properly introduce self to others, ways to broaden interests, how to stand, walk, move accordingly, increase of verbal speaking, using a correct tone of voice, how to sit still, reduction of sensory supports, increase of facial expressions to accurately identify happy, sad, mad and scared, increase beginning, middle, end type conversations, whole body listening, accepting giving compliments "appropriately," increased tolerance of touch, using appropriate manners, demonstrating pretend play, and being social and having friends.

Although neurodivergent children may not be aware of the past treatment of neurodivergents in therapy, neurodivergent adolescents and adults may be aware. And many of these practices are still implemented today. Because of this, professionals may need to state at the beginning of the therapeutic process their particular training and how they work towards being neurodiversity-affirming. Some neurodivergent clients will be ready for this conversation with specific questions and concerns they may have about seeking therapy. Others may be unaware of the past hurts caused by the therapy community. Regardless of the past knowledge of clients, the professional is responsible for communicating the goals of this therapeutic alliance and remaining open and willing to modify on behalf of the clients' particular needs.

When working with neurodivergent children and adolescents, the parents are another important piece to this education. Many parents themselves may be neurodivergent and experienced being part of non-affirming treatment and care. Some may be unaware that this treatment protocol was ableist and hurtful. Professionals must be gentle in their approach when discussing neurodiversity-affirming play and social navigation with these parents. It is not our goal to make them feel any guilt or shame for possibly being unaware of the harm of the past protocol, especially if they had sought this type of therapy for their child before seeking neurodiversity-affirming care. These parents are doing the very best they can for their children and often receive conflicting information from others in the medical and mental health professions. We can have compassionate conversations with parents on why we have chosen a neurodiversity-affirming approach and how past approaches may have been non-affirming toward client care and growth.

Professionals may also encounter parents who have a strong goal of changing their child and are seeking a behavioral approach that may be ableist in nature. Professionals need to be aware that this can happen and make it clear that this is not the approach they utilize in sessions. A helpful explanation of neurodiversity-affirming therapy, with examples of client-led therapy plans and goal setting, and interventions based on client interests is necessary when this happens. Professionals also need to be confident in their understandings and trust in the neurodiversity-affirming approach.

There may be parents who are well-versed in the neurodiversity movement, including the past traumatic history of treatment. They may feel hesitant or skeptical of professionals claiming to be neurodiversity-affirming. In this case, involving the parents in the therapy planning while fully listening to their concerns is key. Since professionals cannot know the previous experiences, knowledge of past therapies, and other information from their potential clients and their parents, it can be helpful to have a checklist of questions to ask during initial sessions. These questions can be asked to both the child and the parents. Possible questions to ask the child and adolescent clients include:

- Have you been to counseling before? Tell me about it.
- If you have been to therapy before, did you feel understood by the therapist?
- How so or how not?
- What do you like about being neurodivergent? How can we bring this into your sessions?
- Is there anything you do that you feel you shouldn't? Why do you think this?
- Can we process this to see if it really is a "shouldn't" or maybe instead something a neurotypical thinks is wrong?

- What is a possible goal you may want for counseling? Some children/teens want to work on making friends, feeling less anxious, getting through school, and more.
- I want to make sure this is a goal you want to work on, not that you think you "should" work on.
- What are the strengths you have?
- How can I best be your advocate? What are things I can teach your parents, teachers, etc. that you believe will help them understand you better?

Possible questions to ask the parents of neurodivergent clients are:

- Has your child been to counseling before? Tell me about it.
- Tell me more about your child's neurodivergence. What are the strengths you have noticed? What are some challenges?
- Do you believe adults in their lives have been affirming? Tell me more about this?
- Do you believe adults in their lives have been trying to change them? In what ways? How has your child handled this?
- What do you like about your child's neurodivergence? What has been challenging?
- Are you aware of the term neurodiversity-affirming? Can I tell you more about it?
- Are you aware of some therapy protocols not being neurodiversity-affirming? Can I tell you more about it?
- May I tell you about the double empathy problem? This concept can help when working on treatment plan goals.

These questions serve as a guide for the professional. Additional questions can be created to ask neurodivergent clients and their parents. The important thing to remember is to have these conversations before therapy officially begins. Acquiring this information before therapy begins helps the professional to be assured that they have presented themselves as neurodiversity-affirming and that therapy will focus on what the child and adolescent clients want and need.

Therapists may have additional questions at this point as to what constitutes a neurodivergent child or adolescent; are there particular attributes common in the neurodivergent population? Chapter 1 highlighted many aspects of this with a variety of vocabulary words, which can be reviewed at this time. There is additional information as to common features within the neurodivergent population. Before reviewing this information, it is important to note that although there are general features that may be seen with neurodivergent children, professionals should never assume that every neurodivergent client will share these features. It is necessary for therapists to be aware of the common features of neurodivergent children and, at the same time, view every neurodivergent child and adolescent as an individual. Within each individual, there may be some, many, or few of the general neurodivergent attributes. Through initial information-gathering sessions, the professional will best learn about the individual neurodivergent child.

The following information comes from Matt Lowry's "The Autism Spectrum" from Child and Adolescent Psychological Evaluations LLC. It describes some key features of neurodivergent people. Although it states "Autism" in its title, these features can apply to neurodivergent individuals in general:

Executive Functioning: Neurodivergent children may show executive functioning difficulties. These include demand avoidance, hygiene, process complexity, autistic inertia, and difficulty changing tasks.

SPINs: This stands for Special Interests. Many neurodivergent children have particular interests in which intense research is completed. Often, this information preference is focused on over mandatory tasks such as homework or household chores.

Stims: As described in Chapter 1, stims are repetitive movements, actions, vocalizations, etc. in order to self-stimulate. Neurodivergent children may show multiple stims and may be getting into trouble because of them. It's important that professionals teach neurodivergent caregivers that stimming is important and acceptable.

Emotional Intensity: Many neurodivergent children have intense emotions and may have difficulty naming, expressing, and coping with them. This intensity may result in meltdowns, shutdowns, emotional overload, situation mutism, and hypo reactivity.

Communication differences: Neurodivergent children may communicate differently than their neurotypical counterparts. This may include echolalia, palilalia, echopraxia, scripting, little eye contact, infodumps, and tangential conversation.

Relationship differences: Neurodivergent children may seek out and sustain relationships differently than neurotypicals. They may show higher levels of rejection sensitivity. They may show significantly more masking. They may prefer virtual friends over in-person friends, as well as virtual events over in-person events. They may wish to have fewer friends and may care less about the age of their friends. They may bond with their friends over their mutual special interests. They may not recall specific information about their friend, such as their name, age, favorite color, and other "small talk" type information.

Professionals can best help their neurodivergent clients by being aware of these characteristics while also getting to know each individual child for who they are. It can be an exciting time for neurodivergent clients when they discover that the therapist is deeply interested in what they have to say. Listening and learning from the neurodivergent child is the best way of developing a deep therapeutic alliance between the professional and the child.

Being a Neurodivergent Child (Robert Jason Grant)

I have discovered through the years that the most challenging aspect of writing about my neurodivergence is writing about my own lived experience. The challenge of capturing a life lived as a neurodivergent person in a few paragraphs or a cleanly crafted essay seems impossible. Perhaps some of the issue is that I do not stop and think about myself as a neurodivergent person in my day-to-day movement. I simply think of myself as me. Much of how I experience the world and navigate environments as a neurodivergent person seems natural and an intrinsic part of how I identify myself. I don't consciously pause and think, "This is neurodivergent me or my sensory areas being challenged and that comes from this place, and this is how I process, etc." Of course, I am aware when my sensory or social differences become needs, and I need to support or advocate for myself. As an adult, this is a component of my self-care, and the autonomy to have control of my environment has been a huge regulating piece that was not present in my childhood.

As a youth, I was completely unaware of my neurodivergence. I highly doubt anyone in my vicinity understood or had heard of neurodiversity, sensory processing disorder, highly sensitive child, or anything related to neurodivergence. As a result, there were a lot of challenges. Things quickly merged into a mix of trauma response, social anxiety, and sensory challenges. With little information provided to understand my system, I took on several negative messages. "I was definitely weird." "I was not like the others, there was something different about me." "I could not do things other people could do." Over time, this just became the norm. I was not the same, and that was the way it was. I was a bright child, so I quickly developed "skill" in masking and maneuvering to place myself in scenarios where I could navigate the best and feel the safest and most regulated.

Much of my youth was about what I needed to do on a daily or weekly basis to survive. My unaddressed issues wreaked havoc on me, especially when I would leave my home. My social experiences were anxiety-producing and my sensory system was constantly being aggravated. I would become dysregulated (overwhelmed and anxious), and I had no real awareness about why these things were happening except I was different and "messed up." School was the worst environment, and I can clearly remember coming up with strategy after strategy to try and get through each day, week, and year with as little dysregulation to my system as possible.

I became very talented at faking being sick. I knew how to make the old-time thermometers (the ones you placed in your mouth under your tongue) indicate a temperature even though I did not have one. I could make myself vomit, and I could put on a great performance of looking very ill. I spent a few years developing different systems for skipping school. At school, I knew all the tricks to spend a considerable amount of time in the school nurse and/or counselor's office (both a reprieve from the social and sensory stressors). I also knew several techniques to get sent home. I developed what I call survival lying. I could and would lie to gain safety. A look back on most of my school years seems sad. I can reflect upon a desperate child who did not understand his system; his system was struggling, and there was little to no awareness or support for what was happening.

My family cared about me; they were good parents in many ways. They had no awareness or insight for what was happening with me, and as a result, they often placated and enabled me. Much of this was due to not knowing what was going on or how to help me. They often responded by leaving me alone in my house, in my room, letting me do whatever was my thing to do that felt good for me. Most of my "happy" times were when I felt peace – when my system felt calm and I did not have to think, strategize, or force myself to navigate. These times occurred most often when I was alone. I sought out being alone; it was safer; it was an escape.

Social navigation was very difficult, especially at school. I was different, and my differences were often not accepted. They were spotlighted and ridiculed. I experienced a great deal of bullying for simply trying to navigate as myself. I begin to construct as much control as I could over my social environment. This meant avoiding all the social interactions that I could. I did not start out as the most social child to begin with. I did not seem to need or desire the same level of social interaction and relationship that others around me wanted. This, paired with my social "differences," created a lot of social rejection for me. Groups were the ultimate nightmare. If I was going to have any social success, it was always one on one, groups were a disaster and often ended in some combination of ridicule, shaming, and rejection.

Things begin to change for me in high school. By 9th grade, the public school became unbearable, and my parents realized this. I could no longer attend. I was taken out of the public school and placed in a small private Christian-based school. There were approximately 15 kids in the high school. It was self-paced, individual learning, and each child had their own private cubicle. This was all a welcome for my system. I maneuvered far better from a sensory standpoint in this environment. Once I felt safe and my social anxiety subsided, I also navigated much better socially. Everything was less and much more tolerable. It also helped that the kids my age in the school were very affirming. They did not reject, avoid, question, or judge my odd maneuvering and anxiety-based responses. They accepted me, and they reached out and offered genuine friendship. This was huge for my growth. This also paralleled an adult professional coming into my life who was also affirming. When I say affirming, I do not mean they all studied and understood a neurodiversity-affirming approach. They probably had never heard of those terms. I mean, they provided an affirming relationship with me, and that made a huge difference. It was the beginning of turning my journey from a survival focus to a healing and empowerment focus.

These later years of high school were an interesting journey. I had discovered a level of social acceptance that I had not previously experienced. I also found myself in an environment that was far less triggering of my sensory needs. I still did not understand what was happening with my system, and I had no awareness of neurodivergence. I also begin to master the fine art of masking. I felt more comfortable by still being masked. I masked a lot. It did not feel safe to let the mask down. Masked often with my peers. I began to understand better what others wanted to see, and I learned how to give it to them despite the pain it was causing me. This is a difficult time to reflect on, as I now understand the negative effects on my life (even today) of the intense masking I performed. It also makes me question the authenticity of my "affirming" late high school years. Did I really encounter these affirming peers who were accepting of me, or did they really never see me and were accepting of the mask? We can ascertain that it is probably a little of both.

I'm not sure how I got to college. It really does not make sense considering the condition I was in when I left high school. The social struggles paired with a lack of understanding of what was happening with me don't seem to lend themselves to college-bound. I will assume this next step was God's guidance getting me where I needed to go. As I entered college, I began to explore more about my system. I continued to grow in confidence and made improvements in my self-worth. I continued to mask and maneuver myself strategically to avoid situations that might be problematic. This meant I continued to avoid many things, continued to implement survival lying, and generally missed out on things in retrospection that I wish I had done. In graduate school, I randomly happened upon sensory processing disorder and the work of Dr. Jean Ayres. The more I learned, the more I felt like I was understanding my childhood and myself for the first time. I had the opportunity to complete some sensory assessments and better understand my sensory profile. I had a term, a description, a diagnosis, and explanations for why many things were different or bothersome for me. It became a cathartic awareness.

I learned that visually I was a sensory avoidant. This is why lighting was a challenge for me. The natural sunlight, especially hitting at certain angles, was painful, even causing headaches. The lighting in certain rooms was also irritating and distracting. Fast and large amounts of movement in my visual could be disorienting and make me feel nauseated. I learned that I was tactile-seeking. This is why I always wanted (needed) to touch everything. If I saw it, I wanted to feel it. It is also why certain types of clothing or clothing on my skin in a certain way felt satisfying.

I learned that I had vestibular needs. This is why I disliked roller coasters and other rides that lifted me off the ground, dangled my legs, removed me from a sense of grounding, or spun my body in some way. They would make me sick, give me vertigo, and create an unbalanced state in my body. This could also happen with certain games and other activities. I also learned that when other system needs were weak – I was hungry, tired, sick, or one of my main sensory needs was being bombarded, then other sensory needs emerged that normally were not an issue. Suddenly noises became extra loud, and I would crave pressure and contained spaces.

I also learned how my sensory differences could affect my social navigation and how the accumulation or sensory, social anxiety, trauma, and other childhood experiences manifested in ways that made me navigate differently. This knowledge became informative and somewhat empowering for me, but it wasn't affirming. I now had a disorder that was the cause, but I didn't have a neurodivergent identity. Many experiences began to make sense and I began to understand how to support myself better and address my sensory needs in ways that decreased my dysregulation. It was a period of time that moved me forward, but my work was not done.

As an adult, I began to realize I had sensory strengths and began to understand how my strengths could be useful for me. Much of my adult years were productive in understanding myself. I grew in understanding of my sensory differences; I discovered my highly sensitive personal identity; I discovered neurodiversity and my own neurodivergence. I discovered my identity. Feeling comfortable with myself, my system, and my neurotype and becoming passionate about helping neurodivergent children become the focus and continues to be the focus.

Today, I am committed to providing neurodiversity-affirming processes in my mental health care practice. I utilize play therapy and help children and families understand sensory differences and neurodivergence. I have often reflected on what it would have meant for me to have had a neurodiversity-affirming play therapist in my youth, maybe participate in a group. I can only speculate, but I believe it would have made a huge impact, especially in valuing my neurodifferent self. Today, we have the opportunity to provide for children what was not understood for me. This is the way I strive to help neurodivergent children feel accepted, value their differences, and strengthen their self-worth.

Being a Neurodivergent Child (Tracy Turner-Bumberry)

Like Robert, I had no knowledge that I was neurodivergent. I was born in late 1969 and was educated in the 1970s and 1980s. I lived in the Midwest of the United States and was the middle child of a father and mother in a working-class family. Of significance, my older sister was only 13 months older than me. We were often compared in school settings, but never at home. My parents treated us as unique individuals. I also had a brother who was six years younger than me.

I was a quirky child growing up, with a lot of energy. My parents expressed that from the time I woke up until I went to bed, I was a very happy child, but very hyper. They felt I was always on the go, and it was difficult keeping me content and calm. They also noticed something that I now know is called hyperlexia. My mom recounts hearing me talking in my bedroom, but it didn't sound like a conversation. She came into the bedroom and discovered that I was reading a book out loud. I was only three years old at the time and was not attending daycare or any school setting, so she assumed I may have been making up the story in my head. When she came closer to me, she discovered I was actually reading the entire book without having any formal reading training. My family was shocked by this and wasn't sure how to handle my reading ability. They took me to the library often, where I would devour chapter books in a day or two. By the time I entered Kindergarten, I was tested at an 8th-grade reading level.

Despite this gift, I had some major educational challenges. The first was that I was left-handed and didn't have any other lefties in my family. What was seen as simple tasks, such as tying shoes, cutting with scissors, and throwing a ball, were very confusing to me. I never knew which hand to use, and since all right-handed people were teaching me, I had great difficulty learning how to manipulate my hands in the same way. I had a Kindergarten teacher who was, for lack of a better word, simply awful. She seemed very upset that I already knew how to read and that I was a hyperchild. She would daily make fun of me by telling the class things such as how I was so smart, yet I couldn't even tie my shoe. She would not allow me to cut with my left hand and forced me to use my right. She would then laugh when I was unable to cut straight. During reading time, she made me put my head down and rest. This felt like torture to me. I vividly remember thinking that I couldn't hold my head down one second longer. This would lead to panic until I figured out a way to cope. I would imagine stories in my head where my teacher was a real witch, and if I put my head up, she would turn me into a frog. These imaginative stories helped me cope and endure reading time while reducing severe anxiety.

In elementary school, I continued to have great difficulty sitting still. I excelled in reading, writing, social studies, and science, but had great difficulty in math and art. I had been tested in school, and it was deemed that I was gifted and needed to skip a grade or two. They didn't see my math challenge as a learning disability or my art challenge as a fine motor difficulty, but instead thought I was lazy and not trying in those subjects. My parents decided not to have me skip any grades since that would make both my sister and I uncomfortable. With her being a year older than me, they believed it would be odd to be in the same grade as her or even a grade above her. So, I stayed in my grade, was not enriched in the classes in which I excelled, and was not given intervention in the classes in which I struggled. My mom has shared with me that going to parent-teacher conferences was awful for her. She was told that I was incredibly bright but lazy and way too hyper. Often, she was told to lower my sugar intake or to make sure I got enough exercise. My mom was well aware of how she fed us healthy meals and knew I was getting plenty of movement. I was very active and would spend evenings and weekends outside, riding my bike, running around the neighborhood, and literally climbing trees! She had recently expressed to me that she felt lost and confused. She would also get very angry since I would constantly be compared to my sister who was a year older. My sister was bright and on grade level in all subjects. She was quiet, calm, and a rule-follower. The teachers loved her. My mom was uncomfortable with how teachers would praise my sister and then disparage me and my abilities. My mom is a shy person, however, so she would listen to the teachers and not respond.

High school and beyond were better experiences for me. I was able to move around much more, given frequent breaks, and took classes with more hands-on activities. I don't recall many negative experiences from this point on and am thankful that I was able to experience some school happiness and success.

Throughout my life, social navigation has been relatively easy for me. I really like people and enjoy talking to them and learning their stories. I had a small group of steady friends and don't remember instances of bullying. I was a strong-willed child, so often advocated on behalf of students who were bullied. I do remember having to really work hard on not interrupting my friends and not always taking charge. I could sense that I was often "a bit much," so I worked hard to contain myself. I loved being alone and often chose to play outside on my own rather than play with my friends. I loved making up plays and various stories in my head and then acting them out during recess. I do remember adults being concerned with my individual play and often called it "isolating." I never viewed it like that; I simply had moments where I loved to interact and moments when I loved being alone. Even in adulthood, I seem to confuse people by my need and enjoyment of alone time. I've often had people express their surprise at how extroverted I seem, but how often I hang out by myself. This doesn't seem like a disconnect to me; I enjoy people but am recharged by being alone. It is something I continue to navigate, finding the time I need to recharge.

The biggest obstacles I had growing up, which I still navigate, were sensory ones. Not much was known about sensory processing disorder, so there were no ideas as to what my struggles were. I had major sensory reactions to textures, sounds, and smells. I would become extremely dysregulated, which could lead to panic attacks. As an adult, I was diagnosed with panic disorder, which is when I realized panic attacks had a definite sensory trigger. I can now prevent panic attacks by always having various sensory items available, but I did not have this as a child or teen. I remember becoming overwhelmed in school by particular smells and sounds and feeling the need to run away. Since I could not do this, I would experience a panic attack and must put my head down to avoid passing out. Some of my teachers were understanding of this and allowed me to go to the rest room or the office, while others were not. I cannot adequately express the shame I felt having panic attacks in public settings without being able to get to a private place.

As an adult, I now know that I have ADHD, hyperlexia, and sensory processing disorder. I can successfully navigate these through many preventative activities such as meditation, movement, being out in nature, built-in breaks, solo vacation times, and more. I always carry with me sensory items to help if I encounter one of my many sensory triggers. I do feel very sad for the little girl I was and wish I would have had some understanding and appropriate interventions. I believe my parents did the very best they could, having no knowledge of what my struggles actually were. I believe most of my teachers were also doing the best they could, but I did have a few that were disparaging and unkind, which I will never understand. My goal now as a neurodiversity-affirming therapist is to be the best advocate I can possibly be for my clients and educate as many as I can on how to best meet the needs of neurodivergent children.

References

Raisingchildren.net.au. (2022, August 15). Neurodiversity and neurodivergence: A guide for families. *raisingchildren.net.au*. https://raisingchildren.net.au/guides/a-z-health-reference/neurodiversity-neurodivergence-guide-for-families

The Children Guide. (2023, November 8). Understanding neurodiversity in children. *The Children's Guide*. https://childrensguild.org/understanding-neurodiversity-in-children/

Chapter 3

Neurodiversity-Affirming Play and Social Navigation

Play the Neurodivergent Way

Play is not work; it holds a natural, intrinsic value (Landreth, 1991). Play performs an important preventative function in the lives of children and serves as an intervention to assist children in coping with personal challenges. Research continues to demonstrate that play performs an important role in the development of the brain – rehearsing behaviors, creating neural connections, learning to problem-solve, and developing creativity (Taylor, 2019). Play is fun for a child and often gives them a feeling of self-worth and connection to others. Unfortunately, play is sometimes misunderstood by adults who work with children. Play can be seen as silly, meaningless, a waste of time, and is often taken away in place of something "more important" or withheld as a reward for some type of compliance.

Adults sometimes make the mistake of assuming children play just to pass the time. This is not true. In fact, children gain most of their skills through playing. Play is how they explore and learn about the world around them. Play should be encouraged for children because new skills are learned by playing. While a child is exploring their world through play, a whole avenue of development emerges for the child. It is important for adults to recognize this and to reinforce play and designated play experiences. Play should be part of children's daily schedules. It should be a priority and allowed no matter how the child's day has been. Play should not be withheld due to a bad day at school or ignored due to a busy lifestyle. Play can be found in every culture around the world. It is well understood that if given the opportunity, children will play, and through their play, they will enjoy, express, explore, learn, heal, and process.

Play is the natural language of all children (this includes neurodivergent children). Playing is a fundamental part of childhood, and it supports children in their physical, cognitive, social, and emotional development. Human development and play are extremely diverse, and, depending on socio-cultural norms, some forms of playing are seen as more beneficial or competent than others. When differences in play do not align with a socially constructed understanding

DOI: 10.4324/9781003468370-4

of normalcy, as often happens to neurodivergent children, these differences are generally pathologized and considered faults of the child to be fixed (Waltz, 2020).

Neurodivergent children may play in ways or prefer types of play that are different from most neurotypical children. They may play with items that are not considered toys; they may play alone, do scripted play, have a single-minded focus in their play, etc. Differences do not mean problems. It is important to value neurodivergent children's play and allow them to play in their own way. It is unhelpful to judge their play as wrong.

Grant (2023) stated that neurodivergent children may share some commonalities, but they also represent a wide spectrum or presentation of identity. Thus, they will also display a wide range of play. The complexities of neurodivergent play are not complex for the neurodivergent child – they understand their play preferences and interests and value (without judgment) their play. It is often the adult (usually a neurotypical adult) that finds the neurodivergent child's play complex. This is often coming from a pre-determined and conditioned view of play, and this view is often not conscious to the adult. When the adult encounters neurodivergent play that does not fit the preconceived notion of play, the adult has a difficult time recognizing and valuing the neurodivergent child's play.

Many neurodivergent children display strong play preferences – ways and types of play they prefer and thus do often. They may not engage in types of play they do not prefer. This is not problematic – it's important to understand a child's play preferences and meet them in the play they prefer. Common play preferences may be in the areas of constructive, sensory, game, and technology-based play. Examples of constructive play include brick building, clay modeling, and working with multimedia tools to create art. Sensory play may include clay, shaving cream, scented items, and music. But a preference can be anything and manifest in many ways. The key is to notice and allow the play preference instead of trying to inhibit or change it.

Consider the story of Elliot, an autistic mental health professional who recently attended training about working with autistic children. During the presentation, the trainer stated that "autistic children do not play, do not understand play, and thus, would not benefit from any type of play related therapy." The speaker used as an example that autistic children lined toys and objects up in a row, and this was not play. Elliot raised his hand and shared that he was autistic, and as a child, he played a lot, and much of that play involved lining up objects. He further stated that when he was lining up objects, he was pretending and doing pretend play. This story demonstrates the importance of non-judgment in the play of neurodivergent children. Play can look many ways and take on many forms. It is not the adult's job to dictate what is and is not play.

Another example is based on the author's (Tracy) experience with play. When she was in third grade, she attended a new school with a large playground. She was excited about a specific part of the playground that had an open field, flowers, and small bushes. She spent her recess time making up plays in this field area and singly acted out the various characters. This was incredibly exciting to her, and she continued this every day at recess. Unbeknownst to her, the teacher was concerned that she "wasn't playing and not making friends." Her mom was called and told that she needed to talk to her daughter about making friends and playing with them at recess. This was surprising to her mom, who felt that her daughter was adjusting well and was talking about friendships made. Tracy actually had made friends, but she was far more interested in playing solo and creating plays during recess time. But solo play was not viewed as appropriate play at her school, so she had to adapt.

Grant (2023) stated that regarding play, there seem to be two fundamental questions and possible issues with adults working with neurodivergent children. (1) Does the adult understand the therapeutic powers and importance of play, or do they view it as frivolous? (2) If the adult does believe in the therapeutic powers and importance of play, does the adult believe that neurodivergent children play, or do they believe that play and its therapeutic powers are somehow lost on neurodivergent children? In the AutPlay Therapy framework, the growth and healing dynamics of play are well understood and are at the forefront of the therapy work being facilitated. Further, the AutPlay protocol unequivocally recognizes that neurodivergent children play, and their play is no less beneficial and is no less important than any child's play.

In the AutPlay Therapy framework and all play therapy approaches, play is considered the agent of change, not an adjunct to lead the child to another method but the process that provides change and healing for the child. The benefits of play and the importance of therapeutic play are primary for neurodivergent children, just as they are for all children.

Neurodivergent Play Preferences

When formulating a group, it is important to discover what the play preferences of the group members are. This can be accomplished in a variety of ways. The following list presents several ideas for discovering a child's play preferences. The professional could implement one or several of these approaches to gain play preference information before beginning a group.

1 Have the parent and/or child complete the AutPlay Assessment of Play (this inventory can be found in the appendix of this book). This inventory could be completed during an intake meeting or given to any caregiver who is interested in their child participating in a group. The professional could then use the inventory to help with cohesiveness in group member placement. For group work, try to allow for children with the same play preferences to participate in a group together. Similar play preferences among group members may be an important indicator of the group's success!

2 Ask about play preferences during the parent and child intake meeting.
3 Conduct an observation meeting of the child's play and take note of what they do and what they seem drawn toward.
4 Assess for the child's special interests using the AutPlay Special Interests Inventory (this inventory can be found in the appendix of this book). This form can be completed as an intake document to help the professional better understand the interests of each child in the group, or it can be given in the group for each child to complete and share with the rest of the group. Often, autistic children and adolescents will have a special interest that they like to learn about, think about, talk about, and do. Many times, focusing on and using the child's special interest in play interventions provides a way to successfully engage with them.
5 Ask the child and/or parent about special interests during the parent and child intake. For group work, try to allow children with the same or similar special interests to participate in a group together.
6 Remember that any directive play intervention implemented in the group would correspond with the play preferences and interests of the group members.

Neurodivergent children may have play that they do not display. This might be pretend or imaginary play, abstract play, peer or group play, or some other type of play. Neurodivergent children may not like certain types of play – it may not be their preference or how they want to play, and certain types of play may make them uncomfortable, or they may not understand some types of play. Neurodivergent children will play – play is the natural language of neurodivergent children, and play professionals should meet the child where they are in terms of their play preferences. Neurodivergent children do play, desire to play, and desire to interact with peers in play but may find the experience to be overwhelming.

There is no optimal way to play, and children cannot fail at play. Yet time and time again, play is boxed into neat and contained categories, often excluding neurodivergent children. Think of the times you've heard someone say that autistic children cannot role play or be imaginative. It immediately frames autism as "lacking" when it comes to playing. The therapeutic powers of play reject rigid descriptions of play and acknowledge that it has endless and unknown possibilities. Essentially, play cannot be fully defined because it is so vast. Our role as professionals is to become play protagonists. We need to become curious, rather than dubious, when we see play that we might not understand. And we need to introduce a play-rich environment for autistic and neurodivergent children. (Murphy, 2021). Professionals may also view themselves as play advocates, ensuring that they explain to all invested parties the fundamental need for all types of play.

As professionals navigate AutPlay play and social groups, they should be prepared for different manifestations of play. Neurodivergent children often have strong play preferences, and this is the space they want to be in regarding the play in which they participate. They may not be interested in or willing to participate in other types of play. A play preference could be in art and expressive play, movement-based play, sensory play, pretend and symbolic play, construction play, digital and technology play, or board game play. Additionally, the professional could witness manipulating and exploring objects, examining toys or materials (touching them or noticing them), repetitive play, playing with the same toy in the same way each session, playing out a script from a movie or TV show, playing the scene repeatedly each session, a lot of movement and changing focus in play, isolated or solitary play, coming into the playroom and isolating themselves in play (distancing from the professional and others), parallel play, and playing with objects not considered toys. None of these play preferences or presentations are misguided or wrong. The professional will want to support and try to engage with the child's way of playing.

"Social Skills" and Social Navigation

Neurodiversity-affirming social navigation encompasses a range of approaches and behaviors that acknowledge and respect the diverse ways individuals process information, communicate, and interact with the world. When addressing social navigation needs with an individual or a group, it is essential to understand and promote neurodiversity-affirming processes. Many neurodivergent children get labeled as not understanding "social skills." Often, this is due to a conditioned expected performance, and if that is not demonstrated, then it is assumed the child must not understand and needs to learn/change. Many neurodivergent children do understand social navigation. Typically, if there is a true cognitive lack of understanding or awareness, there is a cognitive issue such as intellectual developmental disorder or a traumatic brain injury. Professionals will find that many neurodivergent children understand social navigation but that societally normed navigation is not the way their neurotype prefers to navigate.

What is considered social (skills, expectations, norms, navigation) will vary from family to family, city to city, region to region, country to country, and culture to culture. It is a subjective construct. It is also an invented construct by an individual or a group who decides what is and is not okay. It is important to remember children should not be forced to perform a certain "social skill" because it is what has been deemed the norm. Much of this is based on a neurotypical construct that has not valued differences or a different way of navigating. To truly understand the neurodivergent social experience requires a paradigm shift in the way social navigation has been viewed (Davis & Crompton, 2021).

Who decides what is an appropriate social skill? From one culture or society to another, social expectations, norms, processes, etc. change. Typically, what creates these social navigation "rules" is included or created by popular opinion, tradition, cultural beliefs, fads, conditioning, those in power, personality, personal preference, and human growth & development philosophies. Historically, "social skills work" has been devaluing and harmful to neurodivergent individuals. Some programs and methods have used the term "social skills" to implement protocols that have not valued differences and forced neurodivergent children to try and become something they are not, which has produced poor self-worth, depression, and anxiety.

Neurotypical-designed social situations can be confusing as the social rules or expectations can vary from one person to another, environment to another, and culture to another. Often there are hidden rules – things that are understood by many in a particular environment but would not be clear to someone new to the environment. Additionally, social expectations can seem contradictory and illogical, for example, telling a child to work on "paying attention to others" and the very next day to work on "ignoring a particular child." Many social expectations involve a great deal of nuance, which can be very confusing.

In the AutPlay framework, we don't use the term "social skills." Instead, we say social navigation needs. Because of the negative connotation and harmful historical practices around the term "social skills," it is better to avoid the term and use something like social navigation goals instead. The term social navigation also makes more sense, as typically, we are helping a child navigate a particular social situation, which can vary depending on their culture, residence, background, etc.

When professionals formulate any social navigation therapy goal, it is important to consider if the proposed goal is really a social navigation need for the child, or is it something else – could it be a sensory, anxiety, trauma, or executive functioning need that is creating social navigation issues? Could it be the child's neurotype, personality, or preference and should not be pathologized but instead worked with and accepted? Could it be that the proposed social goal is not a need of the child but someone else's need they are placing on the child? Other people (caregivers, teachers, random adults) in the child's life, environmental rules, and societal systems may all be putting forth expectations of the child that are about them, not something that the child actually has a need to work on. The professional may do this themselves, such as by stating, "this group of children need to work on eye contact because it shows paying attention and respect and they need to learn how to do this." When actually the children do not have this need, it is the professional who needs the child to do this. The children may feel perfectly fine paying attention and showing respect without making eye contact – it is the adult who needs this from the child (the adult's need), not the child's need.

Harmful Social Skills Practices

There have been instances of harmful "social skills" treatments or interventions that have been promoted in the past (and still in the present). These treatments may stem from outdated or misguided beliefs about neurodiversity and social behavior. These practices and programs have included trying to teach neurodivergent children to act like or become neurotypical, using force and coercion to get a neurodivergent child to produce an acceptable neurotypical social skill, degrading and devaluing the neurodivergent way of socializing, and labeling many neurodivergent ways of social navigation as deficits and disorders. When implementing AutPlay groups, consider and avoid the following harmful practices:

Aversive Techniques: Some outdated interventions used aversive techniques such as punishment or negative reinforcement to discourage undesirable social behaviors. These techniques can be psychologically damaging and may lead to increased anxiety, low self-esteem, and other adverse outcomes.

Forced Compliance: In some cases, individuals, particularly children, may have been pressured to conform to neurotypical social norms through forced compliance. This approach fails to acknowledge and respect the individual's unique neurodiversity and can lead to feelings of alienation and distress.

Conversion Therapies: Conversion therapies, which aim to change an individual's neurodivergent traits or identity to fit into neurotypical standards, are not only ineffective but also harmful. These therapies can cause significant psychological harm and perpetuate stigma and discrimination against neurodivergent individuals.

Social Skills Training with a Focus on Masking: Some social skills training programs emphasize teaching neurodivergent individuals to mimic neurotypical behaviors, known as masking, in an attempt to fit in socially. While masking may help individuals navigate certain social situations, it can also be exhausting and detrimental to mental health, leading to feelings of inauthenticity and burnout.

Isolation or Segregation: Historically, neurodivergent individuals, particularly those with more severe disabilities, have been isolated or segregated from mainstream society, often in institutional settings. This approach deprives individuals of meaningful social interactions and opportunities for personal growth and development.

Quack Therapies: There have been cases of unregulated or pseudoscientific therapies marketed as social skills treatments for neurodivergent individuals. These "quack" therapies often lack empirical support and may exploit vulnerable individuals and their families.

Blaming the Individual: In some instances, neurodivergent individuals may be blamed or stigmatized for their social difficulties, rather than receiving appropriate support and understanding. This can exacerbate feelings of shame, isolation, and low self-worth.

Historically, in research and writings, any social navigation that has not been viewed as neurotypical has been labeled as a deficit. The term deficit has been hurtful to many neurodivergent individuals who have different ways and preferences of navigating socially. The term deficit implies they are less than, problematic, wrong, and need changing to be correct. The term deficit is also not accurate. A different way of doing something, a preference for how to do something, is not the same thing as a deficit. Neurodivergent individuals may have a social need they want help with or need to address; this is not the same thing as a deficit. It is important to try and avoid using the word deficit and instead use the language of social need. When implementing AutPlay groups, professionals will want to take care to avoid labeling needs as deficits and take care to distinguish between a social preference or difference and a social need.

Some Examples for Application

If a neurodivergent individual does not want to make direct eye contact when speaking to another person, this is not a deficit in social skills; it is a preference or a difference from someone who wants to make eye contact. It is not a problem that needs to be addressed therapeutically. Eye contact is not an appropriate indication of listening.

If a neurodivergent adolescent does not want to join a social club and wants to stay home on the weekend and relax in their room, this is not a social deficit, it is a preference for how they like to interact socially and what they do not like.

If a neurodivergent child does not understand safety awareness in social situations, this is a social navigation need that could be addressed therapeutically. It is not a preference or a difference; it is something that could harm the child.

If a neurodivergent adolescent in a group or with peers is consistently calling the other peers names and telling them they are stupid because they all like Minecraft and he does not, this is a social navigation need in perspective taking that can be addressed therapeutically. It is not a preference; it is a need to understand they can dislike it, and it is okay if others like it.

Jaswal and Akhtar (2019) argued that the assumption that behavioral differences between autistic and non-autistic people that appear to indicate a lack of social interest actually do indicate a lack of social interest and has had unfortunate consequences for how some findings in autism science are interpreted and for what the targets of intervention in autism have traditionally been. They summarized these dangerous consequences as follows:

1 In research, the assumption leads to bias in interpreting and analyzing results (researchers "see" what they expect to see in their data).
2 In interventions, organic autistic behaviors and communication methods are targeted for reduction or elimination since they are considered "meaningless" and/or indicators of social disinterest. The communicative functions of such behaviors are ignored or misunderstood. Logically, such an approach might decrease, discourage, or demotivate autistic social connections.

3 In "real life," trying to insist that autistic people adopt non-autistic communication behaviors may in fact make it more – not less – difficult, and less – not more – motivating for autistic people to communicate.

The implications of Jaswal and Akhtar's reinterpretation are significant. Essentially, autistic people become more socially isolated because their social overtures are misinterpreted and discouraged by non-autistic caregivers, family, and friends. As the authors argue, if an autistic individual's unusual social communication efforts are misinterpreted as social disinterest, and if conventional (and potentially aversive) non-autistic social behaviors are insisted upon as demonstrations of social interest, autistic people will be doubly discouraged from social interaction. Thus, autistic social disinterest becomes a kind of "self-fulfilling prophecy."

It's crucial to approach social skills interventions for neurodivergent individuals with caution and adhere to ethical principles that prioritize autonomy, dignity, and well-being. Any program should be evaluated for its affirming evidence-based, respectful of individual differences, and focused on empowering individuals to navigate social situations authentically and effectively. Additionally, it's essential to involve neurodivergent individuals and their families in the decision-making process and to prioritize their voices and preferences.

How Neurodivergent Children May Navigate Socially

Neurodivergent children, just like neurotypical children, engage in social interactions, albeit sometimes in different ways due to their unique needs and preferences. No two neurodivergent children are exactly alike, and thus, each neurodivergent child will have their preferred ways of navigating socially. They will also have their own strengths associated with social navigation. The professionals implementing AutPlay groups will be tasked with gaining knowledge about each member's social navigation. The following presents some ways neurodivergent children may socialize:

Structured Activities: Many neurodivergent children thrive in structured environments where social expectations are clear. They may participate in organized activities such as sports teams, clubs, or hobby groups where they can engage with peers who share similar interests, and there is a more concrete and organized focus within the social process.

Specialized Programs: Some neurodivergent children may benefit from specialized social needs therapies designed to help them navigate social situations and address other social/emotional needs. Therapies like this, such as AutPlay groups, are relational and neurodiversity-affirming focused, offering guidance and support but never forcing a child to change.

One-on-One Interactions: Neurodivergent children may prefer one-on-one interactions over group settings where they feel more comfortable and can focus on building meaningful connections with others. These interactions may occur during playdates, tutoring sessions, or individualized therapy sessions.

Interest-Based Interactions: Neurodivergent children often develop strong interests or passions, which can serve as a bridge for social connections with peers who share similar interests. Engaging in activities related to their interests, such as gaming, art, or technology, can provide opportunities for socialization and camaraderie. Often, online connections provide more safety, less masking, and a better opportunity for social satisfaction.

Peer-Mediated Interventions: Peer-mediated interventions involve teaching neurotypical peers strategies for interacting with neurodivergent children in inclusive and supportive ways. This approach can help facilitate positive social interactions and friendships within mainstream settings such as classrooms or playgrounds.

Online Communities: For some neurodivergent children, online communities and social platforms offer a space to connect with others who understand their experiences and share common interests. Online interactions can provide a sense of belonging and support, particularly for children who may struggle with face-to-face communication.

Role-Playing and Pretend Play: Role-playing games, imaginative play, and pretend scenarios can provide opportunities for neurodivergent children to engage socially in a playful and low-pressure environment utilizing their play preferences. These activities allow children to experiment with different social roles and scenarios while having fun with peers.

Supportive Environments: Creating supportive and inclusive environments within schools, community centers, and other social settings is crucial for neurodivergent children to feel comfortable and accepted. Educators, caregivers, and peers can play a vital role in fostering understanding, empathy, and respect for neurodiversity.

Family Support and Modeling: Family support and modeling of positive social behaviors are essential for neurodivergent children's social development. Parents and caregivers can strive to appreciate and understand their neurodivergent child's way of being and provide guidance, encouragement, and opportunities for socialization both within and outside the family context.

Individualized Approaches: Recognizing that every neurodivergent child is unique, it's important to take an individualized approach to support their socialization efforts. Tailoring interventions, accommodations, and social opportunities to meet each child's specific needs and strengths can enhance their social development and overall well-being.

Overall, neurodivergent children socialize in diverse ways that reflect their individual preferences, strengths, and wants. By providing a supportive and inclusive environment, offering opportunities for meaningful social connections, and respecting each child's unique identity, professionals can help neurodivergent children thrive by valuing their way of social navigation and assisting with any social needs the child or adolescent is requesting.

Supporting Neurodivergent Social Navigation

Supporting neurodivergent children and adolescents' social navigation identity and possible needs requires the professional to be well versed in neurodiversity-affirming philosophy. Without a thorough understanding of neurodiversity concepts (many presented in this book), the professional becomes vulnerable to implementing ableist and non-affirming ideas, expectations, and therapy goals. The professional must fundamentally begin by understanding that not all neurodivergent children have needs with social navigation. Many do not, and many fall victim to adults imposing the adults' needs onto the child while the child was navigating just fine. For those children who do have social navigation needs, it will be essential to identify the specific needs, identify processes for addressing needs that align with the child's play preferences and overall neurodivergent spectrum of presentation, and ensure that the child's self-worth is always being supported and growing in a healthy direction.

If possible, the child should have a clear voice in communicating what they believe their social needs are and what they would like to work on. What does the child want? What do they feel like they need? The professional's job is to help the child get more of what they want and/or need. Considerthis guiding phrase: "I'm not going to work with you on changing who you are, I'm going to work with you on how to get what you want out of the situation." Any child, neurotypical or neurodivergent, can have specific social needs. A child's potential social needs should be carefully assessed and always addressed through a neurodiversity-affirming process. Consider the following three questions:

1 Does working on the social need help the child better get what they want?
2 Does working on the social need address an issue/struggle the child is having?
3 Whose need is it, the child's or someone else's?
4 Does the therapeutic process implemented clearly stay affirming for the child?

Some common neurodivergent social navigation goals include self-advocacy, communicating needs/rights, perspective taking (self and others), self-regulation, self-awareness, the flexibility of thought, intuition, problem-solving, social understanding, teaching how one's body sensations correlate to emotions and are affected by environments, figurative language (metaphors, similes, personification, hyperbole, symbolism, and idioms), building upon strengths, navigating environments using strengths, coping skills for problematic situations, not understanding unsafe situations/choices, experiencing bullying, asking for help, expressing thoughts, hygiene or health concerns, self-worth, building and maintaining a relationship, addressing social anxiety, navigating sensory and regulation needs, and appreciating their ways of navigating socially.

Several ideas are further presented for promoting neurodiversity-affirming social support. Professionals and all adults and systems can foster greater understanding, acceptance, and support for neurodivergent individuals, leading to more inclusive and equitable social interactions and environments.

Training for neurotypical people: Neurodivergent social navigation cannot be discussed or supported without acknowledging that neurotypical people and neuronormative systems also need to change, value, and appreciate the way neurodivergent individuals navigate socially. Neurotypical people should participate in trainings to understand how to dismantle their rigid beliefs about how social navigation looks and work on their own internal ableist conditioning.

Normalize Neurodiversity: Foster a culture of acceptance and normalization of neurodiversity within communities and social groups. Challenge stereotypes and promote the understanding that neurodivergent children have differences and perspectives that should be appreciated. Educate peers and community members about neurodiversity and the importance of acceptance and inclusion. Foster a culture of respect and empathy where differences are celebrated rather than stigmatized.

Acceptance and Respect: Embrace the understanding that neurodiversity is a natural and valuable aspect of human variation. Respect individuals for their unique perspectives, strengths, and challenges.

Flexibility and Adaptability: Recognize that social interactions can vary widely among neurodivergent children. Be open to adapting your communication style, environment, and expectations to accommodate different needs and preferences.

Empathy and Understanding: Practice active listening and strive to understand others' experiences from their perspective. Show empathy and compassion towards individuals who may face social difficulties due to their neurodivergence.

Clear Communication: Use clear and concise language, avoiding ambiguous or abstract expressions. Provide concrete examples and explanations when communicating ideas or instructions.

Nonverbal Communication Awareness: Be mindful of nonverbal cues such as body language, facial expressions, and tone of voice. Recognize that neurodivergent individuals may interpret or express these cues differently.

Social Navigation Support: Offer guidance and support for developing social goals, recognizing that neurodivergent children. Let the child's voice lead and allow them to be the expert on their social needs.

Promotion of Inclusivity: Foster an inclusive environment where all individuals feel valued and included, regardless of their neurodiversity. Encourage collaboration and cooperation among diverse groups.

Respect for Personal Boundaries: Respect individuals' personal space and boundaries. Be mindful of sensory sensitivities and preferences related to touch, noise, or other environmental factors.

Positive Reinforcement: Acknowledge and celebrate the strengths and accomplishments of neurodiverse individuals. Provide positive feedback and encouragement to build confidence and self-esteem.

Continual Learning and Growth: Stay informed about neurodiversity-related issues. Continually educate yourself and others about different ableism, neurodiversity awareness, and the importance of creating inclusive communities.

Empowerment and Self-Advocacy: Encourage neurodivergent children and adolescents to advocate for their own needs and preferences in social situations. Provide opportunities for them to voice their perspectives, preferences, and concerns.

Collaborative Problem-Solving: Encourage collaborative problem-solving and conflict-resolution strategies in social interactions. Emphasize the importance of listening to others, perspective-taking, and working together toward mutual understanding and solutions.

Social Scripts and Visual Supports: Offer visual aids, social scripts, or other visual supports to help neurodivergent children navigate social interactions and address their social goals. These tools can provide clarity and reduce anxiety for some neurodivergent children.

Social Stories and Role-Playing: Create social stories or engage in role-playing activities to help neurodivergent children address social goals in a safe and supportive environment. These activities can enhance social understanding and confidence for some neurodivergent children.

Sensory-Friendly Environments: Design environments that are sensory-friendly and considerate of the sensory needs of neurodivergent children. Provide sensory accommodations such as quiet spaces or noise-canceling headphones.

Peer Mentoring and Support Groups: Facilitate peer mentoring programs or support groups where neurodivergent individuals can connect with other neurodivergent peers who share similar experiences and learn from each other. Neurodivergent peer support can foster social connections, mutual understanding, positive peer connection, and a sense of community.

Continuous Feedback and Reflection: Provide opportunities for ongoing feedback and reflection on social interactions. Encourage individuals to reflect on their own communication styles and behaviors, as well as to solicit feedback from others for growth and improvement.

By implementing these additional strategies, ideas, and initiatives, professionals and other adults can foster more supportive and inclusive environments where neurodivergent children can thrive socially and contribute their unique strengths, perspectives, and talents.

A Strengths-Based Approach

Discovering and utilizing strengths is a neurodiversity-affirming construct that often gets overlooked in neurodivergent children. When addressing any therapy goals with a neurodivergent child, it is not only affirming but also helpful to work from a strengths-based approach. This type of approach builds upon the client's strengths, specifically seeing them as resourceful and resilient when they are in adverse conditions. This approach is client-led and centered on outcomes in the future individual's set of strengths. Stoerkel (2019) maintained that a strengths-based approach identifies any constraints that might be holding back an individual's growth. These constraints can be when the individual must deal with social, personal, and/or cultural issues in organizations that cannot be balanced fairly. A strength-based approach allows for habitable conditions for a person to see themselves at their best, to see the value they bring, by just being them. They can then move that value forward to capitalize on their strengths rather than focusing on negative characteristics.

A strength-based approach not only examines the individual but also the individual's environment. For example, in the strengths-based approach, it looks at how systems are established, especially where power can be out of balance between a system or service and the people it is supposed to serve (Rapp et al., 2008). When implementing AutPlay groups, the professional should focus on identifying and leveraging the unique strengths and talents of the neurodivergent individuals in the group. The professional will want to encourage the recognition and appreciation of the diverse skills and contributions of each group member. Stoerkel (2019) outlined five tips for using a strengths-based approach with youth.

1 Emphasize a positive outcome – Focus on positive and healthy outcomes like self-confidence, connectedness, or having a healthy relationship with family, friends, and their community (resiliency initiatives). Other positive outcomes could be strong character, caring, and compassion.
2 Youth should be involved in decisions – Youth should be voicing their opinions and reasoning for decisions and development for any services/goals.
3 Long-term involvement teaches sustainment – Youth that can maintain a long-term commitment learn how to create sustainable and supportive relationships and how to be effective in the long term.
4 Community involvement – Building youth on their strengths is highly dependent on their involvement with the community (family, friends, neighborhood, etc.).
5 Emphasis on collaboration – Echoing the previous tip is an emphasis on collaboration and utilizing different resources. Youth need to feel empowered and supported to engage their strengths.

When most people think about social navigation goals, they are often working out of one or a few narrow, socially constructed perspectives. Many social strengths get ignored. Many social strengths are not given the same value as what has been established as the best neurotypical presentation. All children (including neurodivergent children) possess social strengths and other strengths that help support social navigation. Focusing on strengths helps children recognize what they already do well, is more affirming and valuing, and enables them to utilize their strengths to address their needs. Consider the following when implementing a strengths-based approach:

What does the child do well? (dresses themselves, is kind to others)
What has the child accomplished? (Beat several video games, learned how to use a tablet)
How can you assess strengths? (Inventories, observations, asking the child)
What can you observe about the strengths the child has? (Plays independently, follows rules, helps clean up the playroom)

These considerations begin to inform the professional about the child's strengths and conceptualize how the strengths can be used to address any therapy needs. It also helps the child recognize they are much more than their therapy needs. Often, neurodivergent children do not recognize their strengths; some may even believe they have no strengths. A strengths-based approach does not only help the professional but can build up the self-worth of the child.

Neurodivergent play and neurodivergent social navigation have historically been greatly misunderstood. Professionals moving forward with AutPlay groups or doing any type of work with neurodivergent children must understand the history (and sometimes current) unhelpful goals of therapy programs and focus on individual social navigation work with their neurodivergent clients. They must also listen to what neurodivergent adults say about social navigation work and assess social needs, real needs – whose need is it?

Professionals should also view the child as a partner in the process and listen to their voice and perspective. Processes should always be affirming that different is not bad, wrong, or a problem; navigating differently is okay. Processes should also include working out of a strengths-based approach. When implementing a play- or social-focused group or individual therapy focused on social interaction and needs, it is vital to check your process and make sure it is always affirming of the person of the child and their ways of being, preferences, and differences.

References

Davis, R., & Crompton, C. J. (2021). What do new findings about social interaction in autistic adults mean for neurodevelopmental research? *Perspectives on Psychological science, 16*(3), 649–653. https://doi.org/10.1177/1745691620958010

Grant, R. J. (2023). *The AutPlay therapy handbook: Integrative family play therapy with neurodivergent children*. Routledge.

Grant, R. J. (2024). *Play interventions for neurodivergent children and adolescents: Promoting growth, empowerment, and affirming practices*. Routledge.

Jaswal, V. K., & Akhtar, N. (2019). Being versus appearing socially uninterested: Challenging assumptions about social motivation in autism. *Behavioral and Brain Sciences, 42*(e82), 1–73. https://doi.org/10.1017/S0140525X18001826

Landreth, G. L. (1991). *Play therapy: The art of the relationship.* Accelerated Development Publishers.

Murphy, K. (2021). Neurodiverse play is the way. https://www.famly.co/blog/neurodiverse-play-is-the-way

Rapp, C., Saleebey, D., & Sullivan, P. W. (2008). The future of strengths-based social work practice. In D. Saleebey (Ed.), *The strengths perspective in social work practice* (4th ed.). (pp. 197–220). Pearson Education.

Reeve, D. (2000). Oppression within the counseling room. *Disability & Society, 15*, 669–682.

Stoerkel, E. (2019, March 12). What is a strength-based approach? (incl. examples & tools). *Positive Psychology.Com.* https://positivepsychology.com/strengths-based-interventions/

Taylor, E. R. (2019). *Solution-focused therapy with children and adolescents: Creative and play based approaches.* Routledge.

Waltz, M. (2020). The production of the 'normal' child: Neurodiversity and the commodification of parenting. In H. Rosqvist, N. Chown, & A. Stenning (Eds.), *Neurodiversity Studies* (pp. 15–26). Routledge.

Chapter 4

Neurodiversity-Affirming Play Therapy Approaches

The Neurodiversity-Affirming Play Therapist

A variety of play therapy theories and approaches exist in which a therapist can choose to implement in play groups. But before we can assess a play therapy theory or approach for affirming qualities, the therapist must start with themselves. Marschall (2022) stated that when a therapist is neurodiversity-affirming, they recognize that neurodivergence by itself is not a flaw or illness that needs to be "fixed" or corrected. They recognize that neurodivergence can come with its own set of strengths that can be fostered. Neurodiversity-affirming therapy is not a specific set of interventions or things the therapist says or does in their sessions. Rather, it is an approach to therapy and an overarching philosophy that impacts how the therapist views their client and the client's experience.

Marschall (2022) furthered that when a therapist is neurodiversity-affirming, they recognize that neurodivergence by itself is not a flaw or illness that needs to be "fixed" or corrected. At the same time, a neurodiversity-affirming therapist acknowledges and affirms that neurodivergence can accompany support needs. If someone insists that neurodivergence is always a strength with no support needs, they are falling into the trap of toxic positivity and not honoring the full experience of neurodivergent people.

A therapist may impose their own ableist beliefs into any play therapy approach and can view the child through an ableist lens, which would negatively influence the implementation of a play therapy approach even if the approach had affirming constructs. Being a neurodiversity-affirming play therapist means embracing and supporting the idea that neurological differences, such as autism, ADHD, dyslexia, sensory differences, highly sensitive children, and others, are natural variations of the human brain rather than disorders or deficits that need to be fixed. As a therapist, you would work with clients to help them understand and accept their neurodivergent traits, while also providing support and strategies to navigate any challenges they may face in a neurotypical world. The neurodiversity-affirming play therapist would strive to create a safe and validating space for neurodivergent individuals to explore their identities, develop

DOI: 10.4324/9781003468370-5

self-awareness, and build the skills they need to lead fulfilling lives on their own terms.

Being neurodiversity-affirming means application. It should be a way of being in the therapy session. The following are some key principles and approaches that a neurodiversity-affirming therapist might use:

Acceptance and Celebration: Embrace the diversity of neurotypes (the neurodiversity paradigm) and celebrate the unique strengths and perspectives that neurodivergent individuals bring to the table.

Person-Centered Approach: Focus on the individual needs, preferences, and goals of each client rather than trying to fit them into a one-size-fits-all approach. Conceptualize what works best for this client based on an understanding of who they are as a neurodivergent person.

Empowerment: Empower clients to advocate for themselves, recognize their strengths, and build on them to achieve their goals. As a play therapist, be willing to advocate for the needs of neurodivergent children and teach advocacy skills to children and their caregivers.

Education: Provide psychoeducation to clients and their caregivers about neurodiversity, including debunking myths and misconceptions.

Accommodations and Support: Provide intake processes to identify any support needed and work toward providing an inclusive and accommodating therapy space. Help clients identify and access accommodations and support systems that can help them thrive in various environments, such as school or social settings.

Strengths-Based Perspective: Focus on identifying and leveraging the strengths and talents of neurodivergent individuals, rather than solely focusing on "deficits" or challenges.

Cultural Competency: Understand that the cultural humility process applies to neurodivergent individuals. Recognize and respect the cultural and individual differences within the neurodivergent community, including differences related to race, gender, sexuality, and socio-economic status.

Collaboration: Work collaboratively with clients. Provide children a voice in their therapy process and work with caregivers as well on advocating for this voice.

Being neurodiversity-affirming cannot be understood without examining ableism. Villines (2021) stated that ableism perpetuates a negative view of disability. It frames being nondisabled as the ideal and disability as a flaw or abnormality. It is a form of systemic oppression that affects people who identify as disabled, as well as anyone who others perceive to be disabled. As with other forms of oppression, people do not always know they are thinking or behaving in an ableist way. This is because people learn ableism from others, consciously or unconsciously. Bias that a person is unaware they have is known as implicit bias. Implicit bias against people with disabilities is extremely common.

Nosek et al. (2007) reported in their study looking at bias that 76% of respondents had an implicit bias in favor of people without disabilities. This included respondents who had disabilities themselves. In the study, ableism was among the most common and strongest forms of implicit and explicit bias out of the ones the researchers tested for, surpassing gender, race, weight, and sexuality. It was second only to ageism. Ableism in mental health care refers to the therapists, theory practices, or attitudes that discriminate against or marginalize individuals with disabilities, neurodivergent individuals, and those with mental health conditions. The following are some examples of ableist practices in mental health care:

Pathologizing Neurodiversity: Viewing neurodivergent traits, such as autism and ADHD, sensory differences solely through a pathologizing, deficit-based lens without recognizing the strengths and unique perspectives that come with neurodivergence.

Ignoring Intersectionality: Failing to recognize how race, gender identity, sexual orientation, socio-economic status, and other factors intersect with disability and mental health, leading to disparities in access to care and treatment outcomes.

Assuming Incompetence: Assuming that individuals with any form of neurodivergence, including mental health conditions, are incapable of participating in their therapy, cannot contribute to discussions, and cannot contribute to making decisions regarding themselves. Additionally, assuming a neurodivergent person with high support needs would not have mental health needs and could not participate in or gain from therapy services.

Lack of Accessibility: Failing to provide accessible facilities, materials, and communication methods for neurodivergent individuals and those with disabilities make it difficult for them to access mental health services and participate in a play therapy process.

Overmedication and Undermedication: Overrelying on medication as the primary approach for mental health needs without considering alternative or complementary therapies, or undermedication due to assumptions that neurodivergent individuals are not capable of benefiting from medication.

Institutionalization: Pushing for institutionalization, residential placement, or restrictive settings instead of supporting community-based living and inclusion for neurodivergent individuals with high support needs.

Stigma and Discrimination: Perpetuating stigma and discrimination against neurodivergent individuals, which can lead to social isolation, lower self-esteem, depression, anxiety, trauma, and suicidality.

Failure to Address Trauma: Disregarding or minimizing the experiences of trauma among neurodivergent individuals, including those related to medical procedures, discrimination, social rejection, and treatment abuse.

Exclusion from Research and Decision-Making: Excluding neurodivergent individuals from research studies, policy-making processes, and decision-making regarding their own care, leading to a lack of representation and consideration of their needs.

Stereotyping and Patronizing Attitudes: Using patronizing or infantilizing language or making assumptions about the capabilities or preferences of individuals with disabilities rather than treating them as autonomous individuals with agency and dignity.

Addressing ableism within ourselves is the first step to addressing it in mental health care. This requires an ongoing commitment to learn and check for our own ableist thinking. It also requires a dedication to inclusion, accessibility, and empowerment of neurodivergent individuals, as well as challenging and dismantling systemic barriers to equitable care and support. The play therapist must commit to recognizing and dismantling ableist processes and learning and applying affirming philosophy and practice.

Play Therapy

Play therapy represents multiple play therapy theories, approaches, and interventions. The connecting factors among various play therapy approaches include the philosophy that play is the change agent, and the therapeutic powers of play are interwoven throughout play therapy theory protocols. Play therapy is not the same as regular, everyday play. While spontaneous play is a natural and essential part of the developmental process, play therapy is a systematic and therapeutic approach. Play therapy incorporates a growing number of evidence-based practices and techniques to help address a child's mental health needs.

Grant (2023) stated that play therapy can best be thought of as an umbrella term, as there are currently several play therapy theories and approaches that exist. Play therapy approaches range in structure, from being non-directive to directive in terms of the therapist's involvement in the process with their clients. Some theories and approaches of play therapy rely heavily on the use of toys and props, while other theories use toys minimally. Most play therapy approaches involve some use of toys, props, art, music, movement, or games as an avenue to help clients achieve their therapeutic goals. The Association for Play Therapy (APT) (2024) defines play therapy as the systematic use of a theoretical model to establish an interpersonal process wherein trained play therapists use the therapeutic powers of play to help clients prevent or resolve psychosocial difficulties and achieve optimal growth and development.

Currently, APT recognizes ten seminal and/or historically significant play therapy theories and approaches. The list includes Adlerian, Child-Centered, Cognitive-Behavioral, Developmental (Viola Brody), Ecosystemic, Filial, Gestalt, Jungian, Object-Relations, and Theraplay®. Beyond these ten recognized, there exist several established and emerging play therapy theories, approaches, and modalities such as Sandtray Therapy, Family Play Therapy, Experiential Play Therapy, Expressive Play Therapy, Relationship Play Therapy, First Play, Digital Play Therapy, TraumaPlay, Solution Focused Play Therapy, Synergetic Play Therapy, and Animal Assisted Play Therapy, Integrative Play Therapy, and Prescriptive Play Therapy, to name a few.

Ray (2011) developed a list of functions served by play in play therapy resulting from a review of the history and theories of play:

1 *Fun*: The use of play in play therapy provides the opportunity for fun, either for the child or for the therapist and child. Although it is recognized that play is not always fun for the child, especially in therapy, it can often be fun. The allowance of fun in a therapeutic environment lowers a child's resistance to the therapeutic relationship and offers an experience that is often missing from the life of a child who is experiencing several environmental conflicts.

2 *Symbolic Expression*: Play-in-play therapy allows for the symbolic expression of thoughts and feelings. As eloquently presented by both Piaget and Vygotsky, children use symbols for the acquisition of language and expression of emotion and cognition. The symbolic expression of play in therapy invites the play therapist into the child's world. The child is no longer confined by reality and can pretend, creating scenes for the expression of emotion or building of coping skills.

3 *Catharsis*: Play-in-play therapy allows a child to work through those issues of greatest consequence to the child. Nondirected play provides an environment in which the child chooses the direction of effort.

4 *Social Development*: Play not only allows for the expression of the child's world but also promotes communication between child and therapist– or, in the case of group play therapy, between peers. Building and maintaining a nurturing relationship facilitated through play strengthens a child's social motivation and skills.

5 *Mastery*: In play therapy, play is used by the child to control their world. They have the power to be anything and the capability to do anything. They are not limited by real-world restraints. The child uses play in play therapy to develop a sense of control and competence over the environment.

6 *Release of Energy*: Although the use of play to release energy may not seem like a therapeutic endeavor, children are likely to use play therapy as a place of free expression for unused or confining energy. Children who spend the day attempting to "keep it together" in structured environments often need a safe place for energy release, which, once expanded, allows for focused therapeutic work.

(pp. 14–15)

Grant (2023) presented five main constructs that separate play therapy theories and approaches from programs that advertise "using" play or implementing a "play-based" approach with neurodivergent children. The five main constructs include:

1 Play is the natural language of children. It is the way they understand best to communicate with themselves and others. To suppress their natural language is the equivalent of placing tape over the mouth of an adult whose primary mode of communication is verbal.
2 Play is the change agent, not a manipulative tool to lure the child to something else that is considered the change agent. Play is not to be used as a manipulative tool.
3 Play preferences and interests are understood, valued, and, if possible, utilized (focused on) to help address mental health needs and goals. The child is met where they are, with their way of playing (without judgment). The neurodivergent child is not forced to conform their play to a societal neurotypical view of what play looks like.
4 Play is never withheld to gain compliance. Play is not held back as a reward to get the child to perform.
5 The therapeutic powers of play are understood and utilized in play therapy.

Each neurodivergent child and each group formed will have their own individual presentation. Navigating through the various play therapy theories and approaches can best be facilitated through a prescriptive play therapy approach. Grant (2020) described prescriptive play therapy as a therapist-informed method of selecting and implementing a particular play therapy approach that research has indicated is likely to be the most effective for a specific problem or symptom. Created by Charles Schaefer (2001), the basic premise underlying prescriptive play therapy is the notion that all play therapy approaches have the potential to be the one most useful for some children, and no single approach is the best fit for all children. The goal of treatment in prescriptive play therapy is to identify the best possible evidence-based intervention or strategy to maximize symptom reduction and promote overall therapeutic gain (O'Connor & Braverman, 2009).

A prescriptive play therapy approach is particularly concerned with identifying the unique aspects of clinical theory and application having the greatest potential for a positive impact on the target problem or issue. A prescriptive approach does not require therapists to adhere strictly to the initial treatment chosen. Because the overarching goal is symptom relief, therapists explore alternative therapies if the initial choice proves unsuccessful (Schaefer, 2001). The AutPlay Therapy Framework advocates for a prescriptive play therapy approach when working with neurodivergent children. Each child is individually assessed to identify strengths, needs, communication and social navigation style, play preferences, and family resources to guide further implementation of the therapy approach. Each child will have their own prescribed therapy plan implementing methodology that appears to be the best, most effective approach for that child.

Play Therapy and Neurodivergence

Play therapy theories and approaches, especially those with a humanistic focus and foundation, have a protocol that is often affirming for neurodivergent children. Some directive play therapy theories and approaches may need to be more scrutinized to make sure the protocols are non-ableist and affirming. Most directive play therapy interventions are designed to utilize play to target a specific therapy goal or need. Play interventions may involve toys, movement, art, board games, digital play, etc. Although the original intention would be supportive of the child and trying to utilize the child's natural language of play, interventions must still be scrutinized for sending ableist non-affirming messages. The play therapist will need to evaluate if the intervention matches the child's play preferences, is void of concepts that promote masking, stays affirming of the child's identity, and addresses a need without decreasing the child's self-worth. In general, play therapy is designed to be affirming for all children, and thus many neurodivergent children can enter play therapy and feel accepted and valued.

Nondirective (less structured) play therapy holds many affirming benefits. The child is given the opportunity to be themselves in a judgment-free therapeutic experience. They can lead the play (navigating toward their play preferences) and work on, express, and communicate in the ways that work for them. The therapist is attuned and provides acceptance and validates the child's way of playing and being. Although specific targeted direct intervention is not taking place, the power of relationship development, being seen and heard, validation, and acceptance should never be underestimated when working with children with identity needs. Directive play therapy (more structured) can also be affirming. Directive interventions or approaches are typically chosen by the therapist, although the child can be given choices as well. Interventions are chosen based on an understanding of the child and to help address therapy needs. The affirming component has to do with what need is being addressed, how the intervention is designed and implemented, what is being communicated to the child, and is the intervention fundamentally affirming the child's identity (building self-worth) or comprised of ableist ideas, promoting masking, and labeling the child with deficits?

Grant (2023) stated that play therapy has not always been considered a viable approach for working with autistic and other neurodivergent children. In fact, using any type of play-based approach to working with autistic children and/or children with developmental disabilities was considered ineffective and a waste of time. This leading, misinformed, and often harmful belief that autistic, those with an intellectual developmental disorder, and other neurodivergent children did not play, did not understand the play, and play held no therapeutic value for them permeated many neurodivergent-focused "treatments" for decades. Ableist thinking and processes guided many neurodivergent-related therapies, as neurodivergent children were often viewed as the equivalent of an animal that required training.

Today, we fully understand that play therapy approaches can hold many benefits for neurodivergent children and their families, especially in addressing mental health needs with which they may be struggling. Play therapy is uniquely designed for and responsive to the individual and developmental needs of each child, and recently, there has been an increase in child therapy literature emphasizing play as the ideal way to address social and emotional difficulties in children (Bratton et al., 2005; Josefi & Ryan, 2004). Research has shown that neurodivergent children participating in play therapy have gained improvement in attachment issues, social needs, self-regulation, coping with changes, emotional response, and autonomy (Josefi & Ryan, 2004).

On a theoretical level, the therapeutic foundations provided by play therapy approaches of unconditional positive regard, empathy, and congruence (e.g. therapists' use of their own feelings therapeutically as they arise within social interactions) and the method's more recent emphasis on a developmental approach to therapy – all point to the possibility that this modality can enable neurodivergent children to benefit both emotionally and socially. The therapeutic condition of unconditional positive regard concentrates on accepting children's current selves, along with assuming they possess an innate drive towards growth and healing. In theory, this allows neurodivergent children to choose the pace and focus of change themselves, thus enabling interaction to be instigated by children rather than adults, as well as increasing the children's autonomy under the very favorable conditions of the playroom. In addition, play therapy's emphasis on children and adults' emotional responses and therapists' skilled use of empathy to enter children's unique inner worlds essentially target areas of development in which neurodivergent children can benefit (Josefi & Ryan, 2004).

Schaefer & Drewes (2014) presented 20 core change agents of the therapeutic powers of play. Therapeutic factors refer to specific clinical strategies, and the therapeutic powers of play refer to the specific change agents in which play initiates, facilitates, or strengthens their therapeutic effect. The change agents include self-expression, access to the unconscious, direct teaching, indirect teaching, catharsis, abreaction, positive emotions, counterconditioning fears, stress inoculation, stress management, therapeutic relationship, attachment, social competence, empathy, creative problem solving, resiliency, moral development, accelerated psychological development, self-regulation, and self-esteem.

Through specific consideration and selection of the core change agents in play therapy work, all children, including neurodivergent children, can learn the regulation ability, develop healthy relationships, learn how to communicate and express themselves, improve emotional modulation, decrease stress and anxiety, address trauma issues, improve their awareness of self and positive self-esteem, increase advocacy ability, and develop problem-solving/coping strengths.

1 Grant (2023) defined several neurodiversity-affirming play therapy constructs that can be implemented within any play therapy theory or approach to ensure non-ableist and affirming presence in the theory or model.

2 Recognize that neurodiversity means there is no such thing as a "normal" brain. Variation in neurology is natural, and none is more right or wrong than another.

3 Understand that Neurodivergent children (autistic, sensory differences, ADHD, etc.) are not in play therapy because they are neurodivergent. They are in therapy because they have needs such as anxiety, regulation challenges, trauma issues, social needs, parent/child relationship issues, etc. Being neurodivergent is understood as an awareness of the child, which may require different methods of implementing play therapy to match the child's neurotype. Navigate from the perspective: "I'm not going to work with you on changing who you are, I'm going to work with you on how to help you get what you want or need."

4 Honor the child's play preferences and special interests. All neurodivergent children play, and there are multiple types and ways to play. Each child's play preferences should be respected, and neurodivergent children should not be forced to play a specific way.

5 Encourage children's voices to be heard and valued in deciding on processes, needs, and goals. Children should have a say in what needs they want to address.

6 Avoid play interventions that promote masking and camouflaging. Instead, focus on strengths and helping children recognize what they already do well; help them utilize their strengths to address their needs.

7 Respect body autonomy and presume competence.

8 Value and allow for multiple methods of communication.

9 Recognize that different is okay; different is not bad, wrong, or a problem; navigating differently is supported. The focus is never on trying to change a neurodivergent child to "look" like a neurotypical standard.

10 Value relationship development as a core process in play therapy. A therapeutic relationship is key to working with neurodivergent children and their families and should begin with first contact and continue until termination.

11 Understand that play is the natural language of children. The therapeutic powers of play are a grounding principle in play therapy. Play is the change agent and not a manipulative to get to a change agent. Play is not withheld or used as a reward to gain compliance.

12 Realize the play therapy process will involve advocating for inclusion, addressing self-worth, understanding identity, awareness of the social model of disability, the double empathy problem, ableism, and self-advocacy development.

13 Conceptualize that the play therapy process may involve nondirective methods, directive methods, or an integrative or prescriptive approach. The therapy approach and process should be individualized to the unique neurotype of each child, understanding their neurodivergent spectrum of presentation.

The play therapist is essentially the person who stands in the gap between a play therapy theory or approach that may have ableist or non-affirming components and the neurodivergent child. It is the responsibility of the play therapist to ensure that when a theory of approach reaches the child, it has been filtered of ableist ideas and addresses the child in a neurodiversity-affirming manner. Play therapy theories and approaches can be conceptualized as existing on a continuum from ableist to affirming. All play therapy theories and approaches fall somewhere on this continuum. It is the play therapist who recognizes where something falls and makes the necessary changes in protocol or philosophy to ensure an affirming experience for the client. Ideally, it would be the responsibility of the theory or approach creator to scrutinize their philosophy and protocol for any ableist content and ensure affirming ideology is present.

The AutPlay® Therapy Framework

The AutPlay Therapy framework encourages affirming the application of the 20 core agents of change in the therapeutic powers of play. The AutPlay® framework presents the implementation of non-directed play and/or structured play therapy interventions that are specifically chosen and/or created for the individual neurodivergent child. Therapeutic play processes and play interventions are mindfully chosen with input from both the parent and the child. Each intervention could embody one or more of the 20 core agents of change depending on the child's assessedneeds (Grant, 2023).

In AutPlay Therapy, the therapeutic powers of play 20 core agents of change can materialize in a number of different ways. They can also overlap and be integrated in their implementation with some children. Because of the variance in the spectrum of presentation with neurodivergent children, it is likely the AutPlay therapist will experience a variety of the therapeutic powers of play. Thus, it becomes important for the therapist to have a grounded knowledge of the therapeutic powers of play. The intersection between the therapeutic powers of play and the therapist's understanding of the neurodiversity paradigm creates the most beneficial, safe, and healthy environment for neurodivergent children to address their mental health needs through play therapy.

Play therapists working through the AutPlay Therapy Framework with neurodivergent children should take care to meet the child where they are at; do not try to make a neurodivergent child conform to the experiences you may have with neurotypical children. Therapists should enter the neurodivergent child's world – build relationships and try to see things from their point of view. Part of the therapeutic experience is to help neurodivergent children understand their neurodivergent operating system with appreciation and empowerment. Working with neurodivergent clients often means being willing to play outside of the box – to be flexible and willing to go places and try things you might not have done before. While value is found in play therapy theories and approaches, the therapist should never let the theory get in the way of seeing the child before in front of them and being what the child needs them to be.

Ultimately, play is the natural language of all children and holds many benefits, including therapeutic components. Play is also the agent of change that propels children forward in healing and growth. Within the therapeutic powers of play, neurodivergent children have a validating and naturalistic process to address needs and work on mental health growth and goals. The AutPlay® Therapy framework is mindfully infused with affirming play core agents of change that specifically align with the play preferences of neurodivergent children. This creates a natural and affirming atmosphere for optimal progress in addressing mental health needs.

References

Association for Play Therapy (APT). (2024). www.a4pt.org.

Bratton, S. C., Ray, D., Rhine, T., & Jones, L. (2005). The efficacy of play therapy with children: A meta-analytic review of treatments outcomes. *Professional Psychology: Research and Practice*, 36, 376–390.

Grant, R. J. (2020). Play therapy for children with autism spectrum disorder. In H. G. Kaduson, D. Cangelosi, & C. E. Schaefer (Eds.), *Prescriptive play therapy: Tailoring interventions for specific childhood problems* (pp. 213–230). The Guilford Press.

Grant, R. J. (2023). *The AutPlay therapy handbook: Integrative family play therapy with neurodivergent children*. Routledge.

Josefi, O., & Ryan, Y. (2004). Non-directive play therapy for young children with autism: A case study. *Clinical Child Psychology and Psychiatry, 9*, 533–551.

Marschall, A. (2022, November 29). What does it mean for a therapist to be neurodiversity-affirming? *Verywellmind*. https://www.verywellmind.com/what-does-it-mean-for-a-therapist-to-be-neurodiversity-affirming-6829954

Nosek, B. A., Smyth, F. L., Hansen, J. J., Devos, T., Lindner, N. M., Ranganath, K. A., Smith, C. T., Olson, K. R., & Chugh, D. (2007). Pervasiveness and correlates of implicit attitudes and stereotypes. *European Review of Social Psychology, 18*, 36–88.

O'Connor, K. J., & Braverman, L. D. (2009). *Play therapy theory and practice: Comparing theories and techniques*. Wiley & Sons.

Ray, D. C. (2011). *Advanced play therapy: Essential conditions, knowledge, and skills for child practice*. Routledge.

Schaefer, C. E. (2001). Prescriptive play therapy. *International Journal of Play Therapy, 10*(2), 57–73.

Schaefer, C. E., & Drewes, A. A. (2014). *The therapeutic powers of play: 20 core agents of change*. Wiley & Sons.

Chapter 5

The AutPlay Therapy Framework with Groups

AutPlay Therapy Influenced Groups

Implementing the AutPlay Therapy Framework with groups requires therapists to be aware that all participants will have a varying level of comfort with entering groups and engaging in play-based games and activities with their peers. This would be a logical reason that a child or adolescent would participate in a group – to express more confidence in peer interaction, play, relationship development, and social navigation. Emphasis should be placed on understating that these strategies need practice and time to develop. For some children, it may be necessary to begin working on social navigation by meeting one on one with the professional or another trusted adult with the professional. This previous experience of knowing and trusting these adults may help the child feel more confident in interacting in play activities and help reduce social overwhelm and/ or energy drain.

Although this may seem different than a traditional group format, this formation is a group in which children can practice essential skills and confidence-building, but in a safer, trusted space. It also provides the therapist with additional information about the child, understanding their preferences and how their neurotype operates. As children improve in their confidence and tolerance level of social interaction, the goal could move towards joining a group of peers. Professionals should use discretion when deciding if a child could benefit from the type of peer group being offered. AutPlay Therapy play and social navigation groups can be implemented for children across the neurodivergent spectrum regardless of their support needs, but the formation and implementation of the group can look different depending on the confidence, social experience, and comfort level of the group members. Therapists should consider the AutPlay Group Formation Guide (Table 5.1) when working with this population and establishing groups.

AutPlay Therapy groups provide a sense of belonging for children. Many neurodivergent children are left out of groups and activities that involve neurotypical peers. In AutPlay Therapy groups, children can develop relationships, practice

DOI: 10.4324/9781003468370-6

Table 5.1 AutPlay Group Formation Guide

- Decide on the age range and developmental level of group participants. The chronological age and the developmental level should be similar among all group members.
- Decide how many participants will be in the group. Typically, 6 members would be a maximum. A group minimum for a group would be 2 participants. Some of this will be dictated by the developmental level of the participants (the more support needs, the fewer group participants) and the number of adults available to help facilitate the group (the fewer adults available, the fewer group participants). A typical guide would be to have one adult for every two group participants.
- Establish an assessment process to screen for similarities in interests and developmental level. It is better to have a group with children of similar levels and who have similar play and special interests. The AutPlay Groups model provides an intake process to establish developmental (support) needs and a play and social navigation inventory to learn more about each child.
- Establish a screening process to assess for group readiness. Some children may not be ready to participate in a group format and will need to begin with individual therapy. The AutPlay groups model provides a group readiness form.

skills, and have positive recreational experiences. Children and adolescents can gain a feeling of acceptance and optimism about social situations, especially social situations with peers. They may also discover they are not alone and that other peers have the same interests, preferences, anxieties, and needs they do. AutPlay Therapy play and social navigation groups should always provide:

- A safe and supportive environment for children and adolescents to interact. This is always a priority. Children need to know the space, the group, and the therapist are safe for the child to be themselves.
- A natural and playful opportunity to learn and practice social navigation. This must be done in the way that is comfortable for the child, not forced upon the child.
- An opportunity to build self-esteem and confidence in themselves and social situations.
- An opportunity to establish friendships in a way that is meaningful and comfortable for the child.
- A supportive environment for caregivers. Psychoeducation may be needed and provided to help parents better understand their child.

It is important to remember that when working with any child and implementing play or any intervention, the professional will find that they participate at various levels with a child. This is determined by the professional in real-time working with a child. If a child is showing greater difficulty with understanding or feeling discomfort in an intervention being presented, the therapist may become more involved and may lead most of the play or intervention, taking on more of an instructional and psychoeducational role. If a child is showing comfort and confidence in a certain component, the professional will do less directing/instructing and will let the child create and develop in the play, intervention, or group process on their own. The therapist will, at times, be very instruction/participant-oriented, but the professional should always be looking for empowerment opportunities in a child and therapeutically encouraging them to attempt more on their own.

The therapist is the most important component of AutPlay Therapy groups. They are more valuable than any of the toys or interventions that might be used in the groups. Kottman (2011) described the four components of an Adlerian play therapist, which parallel the role of professionals who facilitate AutPlay groups: (1) The professional is both a partner and encourager. (2) The professional is an active, relatively directive detective. (3) The professional is a partner, but also an educator. (4) The professional is an active teacher and encourager. These are certainly roles the professional facilitating an AutPlay group will find themselves experiencing. Children and adolescents participating in AutPlay groups need facilitators who are flexible and adaptable, switching smoothly from child-led relationship building to psychoeducational teaching.

AutPlay Therapy interventions are often used in play and social navigation groups. They are specifically designed to meet a child where they are in terms of their level of play and social functioning. They are also designed with the children in mind, choosing activities they enjoy and want to engage in. AutPlay Therapy interventions can help increase play and social satisfaction as well as other mental health goals and needs such as emotional regulation. AutPlay Therapy considers the variety of possible needs of play and social navigation practiced with neurodivergent children. These reasons may include the neurodivergent child having less exposure to play activities, empathy not being provided by neurotypical children, having social anxiety, and the neurodivergent child having decreased practice in play and social navigation. Often the focus has been on how the neurodivergent child *should* play or how they *must* socially behave, rather than considering the needs and wants of the neurodivergent child. The AutPlay therapist discovers play interventions that are attractive to the client and then presents them in a specific manner so that the neurodivergent child's preferences are validated and they can participate and learn from them while feeling excited and interested in the play.

Children and adolescents are thoroughly assessed at the beginning of group work to identify their play preferences, confidence, and navigation needs and assist the professional in creating group therapy goals. This assessment will also help the therapist in choosing play interventions to specifically align with each child's neurodivergent spectrum of presentation. The professional should implement play therapy interventions in groups using a simple three-step guide:

1 Begin with simple play-focused games and gradually build to more complex interventions. It is much easier to increase the complexity level of an intervention than to correct for beginning above the participant's understanding.
2 Begin with play interventions that seem less threatening or anxiety-producing, and increase the variety of interventions as the group members' anxiety decreases.
3 Try to begin with interventions that are naturally engaging for the children in the group and build to more complex activities that may require greater motivation on the part of the children.

When children and adolescents can feel acceptance and develop confidence in their play and social navigation, they can improve upon a host of possible needs and maintain a healthy self-concept throughout their lifetime. AutPlay Therapy groups utilize play and play-related processes to help children and adolescents gain social navigation comfort and satisfaction. For some neurodivergent children, play can look neurotypical; for others, there may be play styles that appear different than neurotypical play. It's important to remember that play does not have to look a certain way; play is individualized, and something that may not look differently from what the therapist is used to seeing does not mean it is wrong and needs to be corrected. AutPlay Therapy groups can help children and adolescents gain play satisfaction while simultaneously improving social navigation and other needs. The utilization of play as a modality to learn social navigation provides a natural and inviting atmosphere for all group members to participate.

There are a few things to consider before beginning a play or social navigation group. Autistics and other neurodivergents often favor structure, consistency, and predictability. To help increase positive outcomes during group meetings, it will be helpful for professionals to establish from the beginning some directive standards for the group. These include how often they will meet, when and where they will meet, and how each meeting will be structured. To reduce dysregulation and improve successful outcomes, it will be especially helpful if therapists stay consistent, not detouring from the routine they have established with the group.

Relationship development is a critical feature when working with all children, but especially neurodivergent children. History has shown that the expectation of change for relationships to develop was all left to the neurodivergent person to change and conform to the neuronormative standard. We now know the importance of the double empathy concept and neurotypicals' dual responsibility in contributing to relationship development. This troubling history may create mistrust with some neurodivergents, so therapists must show patience and flexibility in gaining a rapport and relationship with these clients. The therapeutic relationship is a core change agent of play therapy and creates an atmosphere wherein children and adolescents can feel relaxed and confident to work on mental health needs. Therapeutic relationship development can be defined as purposeful positioning and response on the part of the professional that enables the child to feel safe, free to explore, express, and discover what the child needs to heal. It is a trusting process where the child believes the therapist is nonjudgmental, accepting, and can be trusted in the relationship.

Neurodivergent children are often, but not always, anxious and dysregulated by new people and environments. It is essential that therapists embody effective therapeutic relationships. Stewart & Echterling (2014) stated that when children are immersed in play activities, they lose their sense of self-awareness and become caught up in the process. This experience of playful flow with the therapist profoundly deepens and enriches the therapeutic relationship. The mindful process of the therapist to stay present with the child, engaging in emphatic responding, provides an acceptance and nonjudgmental atmosphere, and communicates to the child that they are fully seen and heard. This defines the professional's movement in therapeutic relationship development in play. This process will greatly enable further exploration for all types of mental health goals/needs to be met.

Neurodivergent children and adolescents may benefit in various ways from group work. This may include an increase in their own confidence and how to navigate situations that do not value their neurodivergent way of being. Professionals will want to take note of the importance of understanding each child's social navigation with group goals including specific benefits for each child. Structured play or interventions to address social or other needs can take on multiple forms. In general, some points to consider when using structured play or social navigation interventions in AutPlay Therapy groups include the following:

1 Do not overthink it. It is not necessary to have an advanced social navigation curriculum to implement solid, simple ideas to help children gain in social navigation needs. Several interventions are provided in this book, and professionals should remember to keep it focused on the play, relational, and social goals and not make things too complicated.
2 Do not try to do too much too soon. Again, keep it simple; focus on one need and ways to learn that need. Remember to move naturally with the children. Start with a small step and progressively move forward.
3 Do not make directive play interventions too obvious, formal, or "school-like." Neurodivergent children are likely in environments where the focus is on structured teaching with little play or enjoyment. Avoid this atmosphere in AutPlay Therapy groups. Children will be less interested, and less participation will be achieved if the group's atmosphere is too formal or rigid.

4 Keep directive interventions with a focus on need gains as natural as possible and incorporate it into the activity or play time that is planned. Integrate play and a playful atmosphere. This will keep the children and adolescents engaged and relaxed so they can participate and gain the targeted goals.

5 Try to keep group goals fun. Look for ways to add a fun element to every directive play intervention. Structured play therapy interventions should be enjoyable. The professional should try to keep the group process light and engaging even when implementing limits or providing redirection. Remember, what may be great fun to a neurodivergent group may not seem to be fun to the therapist. It is important to focus on what the clients have fun doing and experiencing.

6 Remember that some social navigation efficacy will be developed naturally simply by having the group meet, even if no directive play interventions are presented.

7 Remember that developing improvements in social navigation takes time. Some children in the group may develop improvements more quickly than others. There is no limit to how long a social group can meet, and it would be expected to see neurodivergent children address needs at different rates.

8 Professionals are strongly encouraged to use the resources section at the end of this book, which provides several publications and websites where parents can find more activities, techniques, and games that can be integrated into AutPlay Therapy play and social groups. Although this book includes several interventions for increasing social navigation, professionals can access more interventions and activities to have a wide variety from which to choose.

Handling Undesirable or Unsafe Behavior

When a group of children or adolescents come together in a group, regardless of whether they are neurodivergent or neurotypical, there is always the potential for emotional dysregulation and possible undesirable behaviors. Handling situations where a child is having an emotional meltdown or having behavior that has become unsafe for themselves or others around them should be done with care and support.

In AutPlay Therapy play and social groups, there is no judgment or penalty if at any time the child needs to leave the group. This may be to take a break and then return before the group session ends; it may mean skipping a session, or it may mean that the child discontinues with the group at this time. This should be at the child and professional's discretion, and parents should provide support as needed. If a child is having behavior that is disruptive or unsafe, it could be helpful for professionals to establish in advance an exit or break routine that minimizes disruption for the rest of the group and helps facilitate a positive return to the group. An example of this could be a code word that alerts the regulated group members to stand up and walk to another room while the professional diffuses the disruption. If a child leaves the group meeting for that day, the child should return to the next scheduled meeting unless another decision has been made.

Therapists should not be disturbed by conflicts that may occur in groups. Some conflict is natural and occurs with all children. Professionals should look at conflicts as learning opportunities that can ultimately help children develop social, relational, and regulation navigation improvements. Some children may have several meltdowns over several meetings. This is a part of the process; the child is learning how to be in an environment that may create anxiety and/or dysregulation for them. Some possible scenarios include adjusting a child's participation time, such as participating 30 minutes for several meetings instead of one hour and working their way up to more time. Having a separate break room available that a child can go to if they are needing a break from the group, adjusting so the child participates in every other group session instead of every session, providing a particular child a one-on-one support person to assist them through group time, or discussing with the parent and child that the child may not be ready for a group and agreeing to see the child individually for therapy and working toward participating in a group.

No child or parent should be penalized for a child's behavior. AutPlay Therapy play and social groups are not only need gain groups, but support groups that are inclusive and never should they be rejecting. Consider the story of a mother and her autistic daughter participating in a "social skills" group marketed and designed for Autistics. An autism clinic was facilitating the group with trained "autism specialists." The mother wanted her daughter to participate in the group in hopes that her daughter's social comfort and navigation would improve. A few group sessions into the process, the facilitators asked this mother to not bring her daughter back because her daughter was too disruptive and did not possess the "social skills" to participate in the group at that time. If a socially focused group is not for children who really need help with social navigation, then who are these groups for? This story illustrates the opposite of what AutPlay Therapy plays and social groups promote. No child should ever simply be removed from an AutPlay Therapy group. No parent or child should ever experience this type of rejection. AutPlay Therapy groups are about accepting, learning, supporting, and growing together. Talking with a child and parent about leaving the group should be a last resort and should always accompany a new plan for the child, such as working with them individually.

Most behavior that will occur in a group will likely be the result of the child being dysregulated. A typical difficulty with many neurodivergent children is easily becoming dysregulated, especially in social settings. Neurodivergent children frequently lack the confidence in skill navigation to modulate their emotions and regulate through situations that are causing them distress. A child could become dysregulated due to being exposed to a new environment, having their routine changed, lacking knowledge about the rules of social navigation in particular situations, inability to appropriately express emotions, shortage of coping skills, high anxiety, sensory processing needs, and simply being held to a neuronormative established protocol that does not value the neurodivergent way of being. Many things can cause a child to become dysregulated, and once the child is in a dysregulated state, they are typically unable to control their behavior. This is not on-purpose behavior, and it requires the therapist to be supportive, not punitive.

There is a time frame before a child has manifested into a full-blown dysregulated state, that interventions may help to provide regulation and prevent the child from becoming more dysregulated. If the professional can identify when a child starts to become dysregulated, the therapist can assist the child in regulation interventions and likely prevent a meltdown. Once a child has crossed over into a full-blown meltdown, there is very little that can be done to stop the process. Most children will need to be guided to a safe place and left alone with no sensory input. Once they have regulated, the professional can talk with them and create strategies to try and prevent the dysregulation from happening again. Often simply providing a break option and/or access to some regulation/sensory materials can help the child calm, regulate, reset, and return to the group. In certain groups, the therapist may decide to complete a brief regulation activity with all the group members, assuming that all of them may feel a bit dysregulated. This may reduce more severe meltdowns later during the group session.

Limit Setting Models

Occasionally, behavior that happens in a group will need to be addressed directly at the moment. This is not a dysregulated meltdown; this is an action happening that cannot be allowed in the group, such as trying to eat a marker or painting on the wall. Typically, it is the therapist who decides what is and is not a limit. There are several limit-setting models in play therapy theories that would be appropriate to use. Regardless of the model chosen, the professional should be consistent with implementation. Typically, play therapy limit-setting models are not pre-explained to children, but in AutPlay Therapy groups it is important to explain to the group in the first session what the expectations are for behavior and treating/interacting with others. The professional should also explain the limit-setting model that will be used and provide examples.

The AutPlay Therapy limit setting model (Grant, 2023) provides one option for managing unwanted or disruptive behavior. The three R's limit setting model stands for redirect, replacement, and removal. The professional may implement a redirect or a replacement at any time, choosing one or the other or trying both. Removal is a final step and should only be used as a last resort.

Redirect – If the child begins to or is breaking a limit, the professional should start with redirection. The professional or parent would simply try to redirect the child to another activity, toy, or object to transition their attention off the limit violation. There does not need to be any dialogue about a limit being broken or that the child needs to stop, but it is recommended to add a simple verbal prompt such as "In here we cannot do that." The therapist realizes the limit is being broken and moves to see if redirecting will suffice.

Replacement – If the child begins or is in process of breaking a limit, the therapist can begin with redirecting the child or begin with replacement. These two processes can be used interchangeably. Replacement means literally replacing what is happening with something new or different. If, for example, the child is smashing a toy truck into the floor, which is breaking the truck, the professional would quickly select another object, such as a rubber ball, and put it in the child's free hand while taking the truck away from the child. Replacement can also be replacing a game that is being played by the child with a different game. Where redirection is the act of transitioning the child's attention or trying to distract the child away, replacement is giving the child a tangible, acceptable alternative. As with redirecting, there does not need to be any dialogue about the limit being broken when using the replacement strategy, but it is recommended to add a simple verbal prompt letting the child know the behavior cannot be done in the playroom.

Removal – If a child is beginning to or in the process of breaking a limit, redirecting and replacement should be implemented first. If these processes do not work, then removal is the final option. The first step in removal is verbally explaining to the child that they need to discontinue a behavior, or they may be removed from the room. If the verbal prompt does not stop the behavior, then removal is implemented. Removal is guiding the child into another location, possibly where the child can be alone or minimally supervised while the child calms. In an extreme case, removal might involve physically taking the child to a more secure location. If physical removal is necessary, then parents should be the ones to physically remove the child. This is done in extreme cases where the child or others are in danger due to the child's behavior, and action is needed to keep everyone safe. Removal may also include moving the other group members to a safe location if the child in question is having severe dysregulation.

Landreth (1991) proposed the ACT limit-setting model in Child-Centered Play Therapy and stated that limits provide structure for the development of the therapeutic relationship and help to make the experience a real-life relationship. Without limits, a relationship would have little value. The ACT limit-setting model contains three steps and can be used when a therapist feels that a limit needs to be addressed in a group. The professional can repeat the three-step model for any limit and use this model as a primary for addressing limits if the group participants seem to adhere to the model.

Step One: A-Acknowledge what the child wants, needs, or is feeling.
Step Two: C-Communicate the limit in a non-punitive manner.
Step Three: T-Target acceptable alternatives that the child could do.

An example of using the ACT limit setting model in an AutPlay group would be if one of the participants is throwing Lego bricks at other participants and around the room. The professional would say (A) "Michael, I know you want to throw the Lego bricks, (C) Lego bricks are not for throwing, (T) you can throw those soft balls to another person, or you can build with the Lego bricks." The limit can be stated very quickly, and the child should be given a moment to process what they have heard and correct their behavior. The limit can be repeated if the child continues with the behavior. If the child continues and does not adhere to the limit, on the third time, the therapist can say, "if you choose to continue throwing the Lego bricks you are choosing to take a break from the group or even end your group time today." It is up to the therapist what the final "consequence" will be. Therapists should try giving the statement that a problem item (Lego bricks) will be removed and then removing the item first, but ultimately the therapist may have to state that the group session will end for that individual if they choose to continue to break the limit. If the therapist has made one of these statements and the child continues breaking the limit, the therapist must follow through and send the child to a break time or end their time in the group for that session.

VanFleet (2014) stated that limit setting in Filial Therapy provides children with boundaries that are essential to their sense of security. Limit setting helps children learn that they are responsible for what happens if they choose to break a limit. The Filial Therapy limit-setting model contains a three-step sequence. The professional states the limit, gives a warning, and enforces the consequence. The professional would make a statement such as "one of the things you cannot do in here is paint on the wall, but you can do just about anything else." This is a simple statement that can be made very quickly. It can be repeated for any limits that need to be addressed. If the child continues to break the same limit, the professional repeats the statement and now adds a warning such as "Remember I told you that you could not paint on the walls, if you paint on the walls again, I will end your group time today." If the child continues to break the limit, the professional initiates the third step in the three-step sequence, which is implementing the consequence. The professional would remind the child of the limit and the warning and state, "We must now end your group time for today."

The Filial Therapy limit-setting model can be very effective for neurodivergent children and adolescents as it is simple and concise. The limit can be stated clearly and there is a direct choice consequence if the limit continues to be broken. This limit-setting model could be used as the primary approach for addressing unwanted behaviors in the group setting if the participants responded well to the model. If a child reaches the point of ending their time in the group, one of the adults should escort the child out of the group and to their parents. There is no need for further dialogue or for the child to have a consequence at home. The child can return to the next group meeting.

In Adlerian Play Therapy, limit setting is designed to enhance the child's self-control and teach them that they could consider alternative behaviors and redirect their own inappropriate behaviors (Kottman, 2003). When implementing the limit-setting model, therapists must remain calm and communicate to the child confidence that the child will be able to follow the limit and change their behavior. The limit-setting model comprises four steps; stating the limit, reflecting the child's feelings, generating acceptable alternatives, and logical consequences. For example, the therapist might say, "The rule in the group is that you cannot touch another person." "I can tell you are frustrated but we need to keep our hands to ourselves." "Other group members are not for hitting but I bet you can think of some things you can hit in the group room that would be OK."

There are several possible ways the Adlerian limit-setting model could be stated. Many different phrases could be used depending on the child and the limit issue. The goal is to work with the child in having the child understand the limit and resolve the issue with an acceptable solution. If the child continues to break the limit, the fourth step is initiated, which is giving a logical consequence. This is designed to encourage non-limit-setting actions. This is ideally formulated with the child's input to establish a respectful and meaningful consequence for the limit that was broken. This limit-setting model is very thorough and is somewhat of a process. It may be too verbal for neurodivergent clients, so it is important for the therapist to assess each group member if considering this model.

Parent and Family Involvement

Social enhancement interventions have been found to result in limited generalization of application across people and settings. Whereas neurodivergent children may demonstrate comfort and goal improvement within a therapeutic group environment, effects are often more limited outside of the group settings. The lack of generalized effects of social and relational navigation may, in part, be a result of factors such as training in contrived settings (e.g., pull-out social groups) or lack of programming for generalization. Thus, to promote generalization of group goals, it is important that social and relational navigation groups incorporate natural stimuli into the group environment (e.g., setting, peers), allow for participants to demonstrate social comfort in more natural scenarios, and provide education diversely and loosely (Murphy et al., 2017).

Incorporating parents into AutPlay groups helps address issues of generalization and provides for more naturalist opportunities to implement and practice relational and social navigation. Parents participate in AutPlay play groups by spending time in the group playing with their child and other children or learning about what is happening in the group times. Parents are then taught to create opportunities between group sessions to help their children implement the play and social navigation they are learning in the group setting. This is in the form of setting up play dates with other children or going to a park or public play area and allowing their child to interact with other children and practice the play and relational interaction they have been learning in the group. Parents participate in AutPlay social navigation groups by hosting a "hang out" time for all the group members every other week. This gives the group participants an opportunity in a more naturalist setting to continue the process they have been learning in the group.

More details are provided in the following chapters on the pragmatics of how parent training and involvement are established in AutPlay groups. The nature of involvement will expose parents to other parents and to other neurodivergent children. Participating in AutPlay groups provides the opportunity for parents to work directly with the therapist and their child to help their child gain relational and social navigation satisfaction. Participation also provides the opportunity for parents to spend meaningful time with their child. It's not unusual for parents to report they feel like they are having play times for the first time with their child.

The design of AutPlay groups creates several scenarios where parents will be exposed to and interact with other parents and children. Parents should focus on being supportive of other parents and children, avoiding judgmental comments or actions, and focusing on helping and learning from interacting with one another. The therapist will want to stress a collaborative and nonjudgmental process to parents, as there could be issues that parents disagree about or behaviors that each parent would handle differently. Any substantial issue or disagreement should be brought to the professional to mediate. As parents participate in the group process, it can expose different issues that the therapist will want to address.

Working with children is going to involve behavior issues. This is expected with neurodivergent children as well as with neurotypical children. Each child in the group will likely, at times, display unwanted or problematic behavior. Parents should not be embarrassed by their child's behavior and not allow the behavior to cause them stress. The professional should discuss with caregivers strategies and ideas presented in this book for handling unwanted behavior and implementing limit-setting models. If needed, parents can also meet one on one with the professional to discuss behavior management ideas. It's important for parents to support other parents when their child is having behavior issues and not be judgmental or accusing. Each child is participating in the group because each child needs to work on more engaging and positive social interaction. It's necessary to convey to caregivers that this is a collaborative process designed to help each child in the group improve social navigation needs.

AutPlay groups ask parents to participate on a weekly basis and implement protocols at home outside of the group meeting. Caregivers should not feel overloaded or overwhelmed with group participation. The professional should discuss with parents how to manage their schedule and what level of participation with the group they feel they can manage. Parents are encouraged to take breaks as needed and work with their child at their own pace. AutPlay groups function better with caregiver involvement. It's critical that parents participate at a level that feels comfortable to them. If parents feel too burdened by group participation, it is likely they will leave the group. If needed, the therapist can meet one on one with a parent to discuss their level of participation and self-care strategies. Caregivers should be reminded that they are the most important relationship in their child's life. Participation in play and social groups increases healthy relationship development between the parent and child. Relationship development also provides the catalyst for children to cooperate more fully with their parents, engage more actively in directive social experiences, and provide confidence for the child to explore social activity and growth.

AutPlay play and social groups focus primarily on helping children and adolescents learn play, relational, and social navigation needs, but an indirect benefit of such groups is the parent support that is created. Caregivers with neurodivergent children understand better than anyone else what other parents with a neurodivergent child are questioning, struggling with, and worrying about. AutPlay groups provide parents the chance to be with other parents, share with them, learn from them, and gain support. The caregiver support aspect of AutPlay groups should not be undervalued. Often, parents are searching for a parent support group to share with, learn from, be accepted by, and generally feel a sense of community and understanding. The support and benefits that can materialize from a group of caregivers coming together and working collaboratively to help their children is invaluable.

Caregivers play a critical role in helping their child successfully implement new play, relational, and social navigation across environments. At times, parents themselves may lack critical social methods and may not have a full understanding of why their child needs to participate in a group or how the process is going to help their child. The professional may need to provide psychoeducation to the parents about how AutPlay groups can help address relational and social navigation needs and how this may affect improvement in unwanted behavior (Mellenthin, 2018). Therapists must be prepared to conceptualize not just the child participant but also the parent as a client and consider both parts of the therapeutic group process.

Ethical Considerations in AutPlay Therapy Groups

Ethical considerations for group processes are not necessarily based in any group therapy protocol but rather on the ethical guidelines established by licensing boards and governing mental health organizations. Professionals should take care to familiarize themselves with best practices and ethical guides highlighted by their specific state licensing boards. The Association of Play Therapy (APT) outlines in their Play Therapy Best Practices (2024) considerations for play therapists conducting group work:

The play therapist selects clients for group play therapy whose needs are compatible and conducive to the therapeutic process and well-being of each client. Play therapists using group play therapy take reasonable precautions in protecting clients from physical and psychological trauma. Play therapists explain to group members, and/or their legal guardians (when the group includes those who are legally under guardianship) the importance of maintaining confidentiality outside of the group, instruct them in methods for doing so and make special efforts to ensure confidentiality in settings where it may be more readily compromised, such as schools or inpatient/residential treatment settings. Rules for the group and consequence of breaking the rules should be clear to all group members. If a member of the group cannot abide by the rules of the group, consequences need to be enforced for the protection of others.

(p. 6)

Further, the APT Best Practices guide highlights information regarding informed consent and confidentiality:

Play therapists inform clients and/or their legal guardian when applicable, of the purposes, goals, techniques, procedural limitations, potential and foreseeable risks, risks of inconsistent compliance, and benefits of the services to be performed. This information will be provided in developmentally (and culturally) appropriate language for the understanding of the client and their legal guardian. Play therapists take steps to ensure that clients, and their legal guardian when applicable, understand the implications of diagnosis, treatment modalities, treatment interventions, the intention of assessment and reports, and fees and billing arrangements. Clients have the right to expect confidentiality and to be provided with an explanation of its limitations, including disclosure to appropriate legal guardian(s), disclosure as legally required and for safety when an immediate safety risk is revealed, suspicion of child abuse or other safety issue, supervision and/or treatment team case reviews, and requests made by the payer, and/or governmental authority and/or by court order to obtain information about any documents or documentations in their case records. Play therapists seek legal guardian's signature on all consents, including for treatment whenever applicable and when not constricted by state and/or federal laws and their legal and ethical codes of their license and professional organization.

(p. 4)

In AutPlay Therapy groups, one of the primary areas to address is confidentiality. Because of the nature of parents' involvement in the group process, children and parents will be exposed to other children and parents and will likely be aware of information about the other children and parents. Therapists cannot guarantee that group participants will maintain the confidentiality and privacy of other group participants. The importance of maintaining confidentiality should be communicated to the group (Sweeney et al., 2014). The AutPlay professional must stress to group participants (children and caregivers) the importance of maintaining confidentiality and that, due to the nature of being involved in a group, confidentiality cannot be guaranteed. There should be a process established by the professional (which should be shared with group participants) outlining the consequences when group confidentiality and privacy are broken. The process of maintaining confidentiality and adherence to keeping information private should be outlined in the informed consent document that caregivers must sign prior to beginning the group process.

References

Association for Play Therapy. (2024). Play therapy best practices. https://www.a4pt.org/page/Publications

Grant, R. J. (2023). *The AutPlay therapy handbook: Integrative family play therapy with neurodivergent children*. Routledge.

Kottman, T. (2003). *Partners in play: An Adlerian approach to play therapy*. American Counseling Association.

Kottman, T. (2011). *Play therapy: Basics and beyond*. American Counseling Association.

Landreth, G. L. (1991). *Play therapy: The art of the relationship*. Brunner-Routledge.

Murphy, M., Burns, J., & Kilbey, E. (2017). Using personal construct methodology to explore relationships with adolescents with autism spectrum disorder. *Research in Developmental Disabilities, 70*, 22–32.

Stewart, A. L., & Echterling, L. G. (2014). Therapeutic relationship. In C. E. Schaefer & A. A. Drewes (Eds.), *The therapeutic powers of play: 20 core agents of change* (2nd ed.). Wiley.

Sweeney, D. S., Baggerly, J. N., & Ray, D. C. (2014). *Group play therapy: A dynamic approach*. Routledge.

VanFleet, R. (2014). *Filial therapy: Strengthening parent-child relationships through play* (3rd ed.). Professional Resource Press.

Chapter 6

AutPlay® Therapy Play Groups with Children and Parents (10 Session Framework)

Play Therapy Groups and the FMA

Play therapy groups developed in part because patterns of behavior emerged in children in group environments that were not present in the play of individual children. Therapeutic and other types of groups focusing on children have grown in the past decade. Professionals have discovered that processes in groups cannot be replicated in individual work, and the group atmosphere holds much benefit for children (Knell, 1997). Groups serve as a practice field for the outside world, and the expressive and projective nature of play groups enable this practice to become real, thus easier to transfer and generalize to other settings and experiences (Sweeney et al., 2014). Group play and/or the implementation of a therapeutic group has primarily been centered on neurotypical experiences. While much has become understood about neurotypical group play and the benefits of group work, little has been researched or understood about neurodivergent group play and the benefits of a therapeutic group experience.

AutPlay framework play groups are based on an integration of family play therapy approaches, neurodiversity-affirming understanding, and processes found in the Follow Me Approach (FMA). The FMA is a more nondirective play method in the AutPlay Therapy framework that is used with children and adolescents who (1) have high support needs, (2) cannot or do not engage in more structured (directive) interventions, (3) may benefit from a more nondirective approach, (4) families that may benefit from a more nondirective playtime approach, (5) and children who are too young to participate in therapist-structured approaches. Play groups can apply to or be beneficial for any aged child or adolescent. The FMA focuses on relationship development, safety, connection, and engagement, and a movement for the child from anxiety and uncertainty to naturally engaging and attunement processes and potentially the ability to complete directive play interventions with the professional and caregivers (Grant, 2023).

DOI: 10.4324/9781003468370-7

Axline (1969) described nondirective play as therapy that starts where the child is and bases the process on the present configuration, allowing for change from minute to minute during the therapeutic contact. It grants the child permission to be themselves and accept that self completely, without evaluation or pressure to change. It offers the child the opportunity to learn to know themselves and to openly chart their own course so they may form a more satisfactory design for living. Landreth (1991) stated that the therapist recognizes that growth is a slow process, not to be pushed, prodded, and hurried along. This is a time when the child can relax, a place where growth takes place naturally without being forced. It is the focus on relationship development with the neurodivergent child that facilitates the child becoming more comfortable and confident, which promotes engagement gains.

The FMA creates space for the neurodivergent child to feel accepted and free to explore and express (Grant, 2023). The FMA is an integration and extension of established nondirective play therapy theories and approaches such as child-centered play therapy, child–parent relationship therapy, and filial therapy. Ray, Sullivan, and Carlson (2012) described that in nondirective play therapy approaches, the therapist seeks to understand the child in the context of their world. The therapist provides full acceptance to the child, offers unconditional positive regard, and sends a message of respect and safety to children to enable them to share their world freely. The FMA utilizes established nondirective play therapy processes and individualizes the processes to the specific neurodivergent child being sure to acknowledge the neurodivergent child's play preferences and interests as well as their unique strengths (Grant, 2023).

In FMA, the therapist and child participate in a typical play therapy room environment. The child is given no directive instructions from the professional other than a structuring statement to begin the session, such as "This is the playroom and you can play with anything you want and I will be in here with you." The therapist follows the child's lead, moving with the child around the playroom and trying to engage with the child in whatever activity or toy they are playing with. The professional lets the child lead but looks for natural opportunities to get involved with what the child is doing. The professional transitions as the child transitions and is continuously looking for openings to connect with the child. As the child transitions from one toy or activity to another, the therapist transitions with the child. This basic FMA structure is implemented in AutPlay play groups.

Throughout AutPlay play groups, the professional is using a variety of FMA skills, including reflecting and tracking statements and being mindful of the child's comfort level. In AutPlay play groups, it is important to not only share physical space with the child but also share attention, emotion, and understanding with the child. Parents also participate in AutPlay Play groups and are taught FMA play skills to implement with their child. Caregivers are also instructed on how to facilitate play meetings outside of the play group meeting. Parent-hosted "play dates" help to further play group goals outside of the formal clinical group experience. The following highlights key FMA skills the professional and/or parent implements when facilitating AutPlay play groups:

1 *Make a Structuring Statement*: Begin the group session with a structuring statement such as "This is the playroom, and you can play with anything you want in here and I will be in here with you."

2 *Follow the Children*: The children lead, and the professional follows the children figuratively and literally. The professional lets the children move around the playroom and allows children to play with anything and in whatever way they choose. The professional makes every effort to attune to the child (staying present), move with the children, sit by the children, and transition as the children transition.

3 *Make Tracking Statements*: These are statements that the professional makes periodically to track what the child is doing. Tracking statements are not a running commentary on whatever the children are doing. The professional will periodically note different things that different children are doing and make a verbal tracking statement. These statements communicate to the child that the professional is present, noticing, and attuning to the child. They also communicate to other children a model of attunement with each other. For example: "John, you are playing in the sand tray." "Alex, you just shot the Nerf gun." "Kylie, you are looking around at all the toys in here." "Kim, you are done with the doll house and now you found some puppets."

4 *Make Reflecting Statements*: These are statements that the professional makes when they notice a child displaying a state of being, feeling, or emotion. These statements are made when the professional sees or hears the child communicate a state of being or feeling. For example: "Albert, that makes you mad." "Tony, you feel sad that there is no more paint." "Sarah, that is making you laugh." "Molly, you are confused about that toy, not sure what it is." For some neurodivergent children, they may experience states of being or feelings in ways that are not the common neurotypical method of expression. The professional should be sensitive to this and try to observe each child's way of communicating what they are experiencing. Some neurodivergent children may have alexithymia, characterized by an impaired ability to be aware of, explicitly identify, and describe one's feelings (Hogeveen & Grafman, 2021). In some instances, it may be better for the professional to not name a specific feeling but speak in more general terms such as "Sam, something is happening for you," "David, something just changed for you," "Kate, there is something going on for you," or "Erin, you are having a reaction to that."

5 *Ask Questions*: The professional should periodically ask the children questions. A question can be directed at a particular child or the whole group. Questions are periodically asked to help promote engagement with the professional and between group members. The professional should try to ask questions that are relevant to what is happening in the play group. For example: A child picks up a basketball. The professional might ask, "Alex, do you have a basketball at home?" A child is painting. The professional might ask, "Kathy, what is your favorite color?" The group members seem to be exploring options. The professional might ask, "Would anyone like to hit a balloon back and forth with each other?"

6 *Attempt to Engage with the Children through Their Play*: The professional should periodically try to engage or play with the children in whatever they are doing. This should reflect a natural process and not be forced or awkward. If the professional tries to engage with a child and the child displays a lack of interest or displeasure with the attempt, the professional should not continue. For example, a child is playing in the sand tray, filling a bucket with sand. The professional might try scooping up some sand and pouring it on the child's hand or scooping up some sand and putting it in the bucket the child is trying to fill. Another example: The child is playing with some balls; the professional might pick up a ball and try to roll it or toss it to the child. The professional can also attempt to have children join each other in play. Again, this should be as natural as possible and never forced.

7 *Monitoring for Dysregulation*: The professional should be sensitive to each child's comfort level, especially regarding attempts to engage with the child and being around other children. If the professional notices that a child is becoming uncomfortable or dysregulated by the professional's attempts to engage, the professional should discontinue making attempts to engage and move away from that child for a period of time and try again later. If the professional notices a child is becoming uncomfortable or dysregulated by being around the other children or from something another child is doing, the professional should have a plan for the child to take a break and regulate. This is discussed in more detail later in this chapter.

AutPlay play groups are typically designed for and can be implemented with any aged neurodivergent child who may benefit from the experience. These play groups are designed with a neurodivergent child experience in mind, but it is possible that a neurotypical child may benefit from the group experience as well. Neurodivergent is conceptualized in general and not limited to one or two neurominority experiences. What separates AutPlay play groups from other group experiences is the professional's clear understanding and value of the neurodivergent experience, and implementing group processes from a neurodiversity-affirming philosophy. The following pragmatics will discuss this in more detail. The pragmatics will also highlight how caregivers are involved in AutPlay play groups, but it is possible to facilitate play groups without caregiver involvement. The AutPlay therapy framework across individual therapy or group implementation is always designed to be fluid and ready for individualization that adjusts protocols to meet the needs of the client(s) being served.

Pragmatics of AutPlay Play Groups

Definition of AutPlay Play Groups: Based on an integration of family play therapy, AutPlay Therapy FMA and neurodiversity-affirming philosophy. These groups are designed for neurodivergent children of any age but may be most helpful for high-support needs of children and adolescents, children who cannot or do not engage in more structured interventions, children who may prefer a more nondirective play approach or a more family-focused approach where there may be benefit from participating in a more nondirective family play time. AutPlay play groups provide an atmosphere of playful interaction facilitated by a professional and can include caregiver participation.

Role of the Professional: The professional organizes and facilitates the play group process, ensuring an atmosphere that is safe and affirming for children. The therapist is a player and an encourager for both the children and the caregivers. Often, the professional serves as a role model and a teacher. The professional is active in play groups by attempting to engage and play with children, fostering engagement among children, establishing limits when necessary, and providing examples of affirming play strategies to caregivers. The therapist is diligent to adhere play groups skills, maintain an openness to any needed adjustments or accommodations, and be an example of neurodiversity-affirming care.

Being Neurodiversity-Affirming: AutPlay groups begin with the professional's philosophy and commitment to implementing neurodiversity-affirming constructs. Being neurodiversity-affirming is the application of the neurodiversity paradigm and movement. The paradigm and movement propose that neurodiversity is real and a natural part of the human experience. Those who are neurodivergent should be valued and appreciated regarding their neurodiversity. Different ways of communicating, thinking, processing, socializing, and navigating the world are appreciated and neurodivergent identity is empowered. In AutPlay groups, this includes supporting play preferences and interests, joining in the child's play, teaching caregivers neurodiversity-affirming concepts, appreciating the child's social navigation preferences, and allowing the child to interact in the ways in which they are comfortable. Essentially, being neurodiversity-affirming means it is okay to be neurodivergent, and group processes should never include trying to make the neurodivergent child look or become neurotypical.

Structure: AutPlay play groups are typically 50 minutes and consist of 20 group sessions. The group begins with a meeting in the professional's clinic where children participate in a play group (this typically occurs in a playroom or designated play space). The next week, the group participants meet together outside of the clinic to have a less formal "play date" meeting. This meeting is hosted by one of the participant's caregivers. The meetings alternate in this fashion weekly for 20 meetings – ten in-clinic play meetings and ten outside "play date" meetings. A step-by-step organization and structure guide for starting an AutPlay play group is provided in the appendix section of this book.

Generating Interest in a Group: Professionals should conduct a needs assessment in their local community regarding offering AutPlay play groups. As neurodivergent children are often underserved, and especially through a neurodiversity-affirming process, it is likely the need will be present. This can be done by contacting local agencies that work with neurodivergent children, contacting early intervention programs, contacting preschools, asking other mental health providers in the community, and checking with local parent support groups. It may be something that can be generated from the professional's own caseload.

Organization of a Group: The professional should decide on a possible start date and location for the group. The therapist should also prepare any forms needed for the group and begin to market the group. A sample marketing flier is provided in the appendix section of this book. It is sometimes helpful to keep an active list of those who are interested in a group. Once enough individuals are interested to form a group, they can be contacted and a start date established.

Assessing/Screening Group Members: It is important that group members are as similar as possible when it comes to age, needs, neurodivergent spectrum of presentation, and developmental level. Gender tends to not be as important as having children in the same group who have a similar neurodivergent spectrum of presentation. When groups comprise many ages and several different neuro-divergent presentations, it can sometimes be inconsistent, chaotic, and create dynamics that make it difficult to create a safe and engaging environment. The Intake Form and Group Readiness Questionnaire found in the appendix section of this book can be used to help assess group participants and form groups that can be cohesive.

The therapist should meet with each parent and child who might be interested in participating in a play group. This meeting is an opportunity to complete necessary documents, understand the child's neurodivergent spectrum of presentation, and decide if the child would be an appropriate fit for the group that is beginning. If the child is assessed as not ready for a group experience, the professional could try to offer a meeting with the child for individual therapy and work toward joining a group. The therapist can offer more than one group. This might be especially helpful if there are children of different presentations wanting to attend; the professional could offer multiple groups, matching the children with the best-fitting group. It might be necessary to place some children on a group wait list until there are enough children interested in participating in a group that are similar in age and presentation. Once group interest is established, the professional should meet with each caregiver/child, have them complete the Group Readiness Questionnaire, and do simple observation of the child. These processes will help solidify the cohesive placement of group participants.

Who Can Participate: Any child can participate if it seems the group would be appropriate for the child and their therapy needs. Participants do not need a formal diagnosis to participate, and they do not need to possess a specific neurominority identity. Although a primary focus of the group is neurodivergent children, any child who might benefit from the play groups format could participate.

Group Size: The typical size of a group should be four to five children, with no more than six. Anything larger will negatively affect the ability of the group to naturally connect and work on engagement and group play processes. Groups can be smaller and still be beneficial, but larger groups should be avoided. It would be better to have two groups of three than one group of six. The minimum number of participants for a group is two. Professionals should strive for a ratio of one adult for every two children, so the larger the group size, the more adults that will be needed to facilitate the group. These are recommendations for group size. This will vary depending on the spectrum of presentation of the participants. It might be possible for one professional to work with a group of three children if they were older children and they all had low support needs. Likewise, if the participants all have high support needs, the group may require a one-to-one ratio of child to adult.

Length of Group Meetings: The length of time a group meets may vary depending on the professional's preference, but the group structure for AutPlay play groups is based on a 50-minute group session. Some professionals may prefer to lengthen or shorten the group time.

Number of Group Meetings: AutPlay play groups meet for ten in the clinic at more formal play times and ten outside of the clinic at less formal "play date" times. This creates a total of 20 meetings. The formal and informal meetings alternate from week to week. The first week the group meets in the clinic; the next week they meet outside of the clinic. The professional does not attend the outside of the clinic meetings; these are hosted by one of the participant's caregivers. It is important to formally end a group after the 20 meetings to give children and caregivers a clean opportunity to leave the group. The professional can begin new groups at any time or start another group when one ends, and the new groups can include some of the same participants from the previous group.

Play Preferences and Interests: Since much of the group focus will be on play, it is important to assess each child's play preferences and interests. The AutPlay Groups Assessment of Play form is provided in the appendix section of this book. The professional will give the parent the play assessment form to complete as part of the group intake process prior to the group beginning. The professional will want to note each child's play preferences and ideally place children with similar play preferences together. This can help facilitate group comfort, engagement, and cohesion.

Social Navigation: AutPlay play groups provide an integrative process of clinical and natural opportunity for children and adolescents to engage and connect with each other. A more formal, nondirective play time happens in the clinic meetings, while a less formal, more naturalist process happens during outside of the clinic meetings. Both experiences are important for neurodivergent children to experience social interaction in a safe and exploratory process. In AutPlay Play Groups, play is the process by which children develop more comfort and empowerment in social and peer interaction. The play process facilitates the acquisition of social navigation in ways that are respectful of the child's navigation preferences. Children should not be forced to interact in ways that are stressful, dysregulating, and contrary to their neurodivergent differences. The

Table 6.1 Meeting Places for Parent Hosted Play Groups

Parent's Home	Park
Chucky Cheese	Public Library
Pet Store	Kids Play Place
Kids Museum	School Playground
Restaurant Play Area	Petting Zoo

professional should always be affirming and mindful of social navigation through engagement, connection, and play that supports neurodiversity differences.

Group Meeting Locations: The professional will likely have in-clinic meetings at their clinic or some arranged meeting place. It is ideal for the in-clinic meeting location to be in a playroom or an established play space and to stay consistent throughout the duration of the group. For the caregiver hosted, outside the clinic play meetings, there are many options where a group could meet (this is typically decided on by the caregiver who is hosting). A common setting such as a parent's home, a church, or a support group meeting facility would certainly work. It is highly encouraged that some of the play date meetings occur in public. This may be a certain event or specific activity designed for children; it may simply be going to a restaurant or park. Some caregivers may need help in deciding where to meet. Table 6.1 provides some meeting place options for caregivers. Also, the therapist should communicate to caregivers that the caregiver-hosted play meetings should not include any formal social interventions. This is a time for the participants to be together and experience natural social play their way. The caregivers can help their child to interact, but there should be no pressure or purposeful teaching. The participants need this time to be with other children and enjoy a group social play experience at their own pace.

It can be helpful for caregivers to understand the dynamics of the children in the group and where each child is in terms of the spectrum of presentation and window of tolerance for certain situations. It is important for caregivers to know of the particular needs of each child, such as any sensory differences, allergies, medical conditions, or fears related to certain environments. Any information about any of the group participants that would guide the selection of a location or event for a caregiver-hosted play meeting should be shared with the caregivers to avoid any potential issues. Where to meet and the type of play experience should be decided on and communicated the week before the parent-hosted play meeting. Typically, the professional will have this information and share it with all the children and caregivers at the end of the in-clinic meeting. This information is included on the Session Overview Form (located in the appendix section) that is given to caregivers at the end of each in-clinic meeting.

Limit-Setting Behavior: The professional will want to choose one of the limit-setting models defined in this book and explain the limit-setting model to the caregivers during the group screening meeting. Modeling and practicing the limit-setting model during this meeting may also be beneficial for the caregivers. The therapist should use the limit-setting model consistently. Each model provides for a final consequence of ending the group time for the child if the behavior does not change and/or is too disruptive. The professional should be patient and implement limits at a minimum. It is expected that there will be some unwanted and troublesome behavior. This should be relayed to all the caregivers, so they are not surprised if something happens. If it is something the therapist can work with and correct easily, then there is no need for further action. Some children may exhibit a limit-setting behavior due to becoming dysregulated with the experience or by being around other children. If possible, providing children the opportunity to move to a location in the playroom and play alone for a while can be helpful. It can also be helpful to have another room available that a child can go to for a break from the group. Providing a break from the interaction can help children regulate and manage through the play group experience.

When caregivers are hosting a play meeting, the professional will not typically be present. The parents may need some brief instruction on how to handle limit-setting behavior. Professionals can teach the caregivers limit setting models and other interventions. It's important to explain to parents that behaviors will likely occur during a caregiver-hosted meeting. If a caregiver has certain strategies they typically implement to help their child calm, the caregiver should implement these strategies. If a caregiver feels like they and their child need to leave the play meeting, this is Ok. The parent and child should leave, and they can try again at the next meeting. Other caregivers should get involved only if the caregiver of the child having the limit-setting behavior asks for assistance. It is important that the parent of the child having the limit-setting behavior is the primary person addressing their child and trying to manage the situation.

Caregivers as Co-Change Agents: Caregivers can participate in AutPlay play groups in two ways. In the AutPlay Therapy FMA, parents work with the professional in learning how to have special play times at home with their child. In AutPlay Play Groups, caregivers host a play meeting outside of the clinic to help further the acquisition of engagement gains. This process is fully explained to caregivers during the initial screening/consultation about the play group. All caregivers are asked to participate, and a schedule is made that identifies which each caregiver will host a play meeting. Any training, suggestions, or help a caregiver may need should be provided by the professional. If a parent has concerns and would like suggestions for hosting a play meeting, the professional should meet with the caregiver and provide the information they are requesting. The therapist should communicate to caregivers that they are an important part of the play group process and empower caregivers to feel confident in their participation.

When parents host a play meeting, the other caregivers should participate in each group meeting as much as possible. It may not be necessary for every caregiver to be at every meeting if caregivers are comfortable with others taking care of their children (this will depend on the size of the group, the age of the children, and the support needs of group participants). It is important that there are enough caregivers at each group meeting to care for the children and facilitate the play meeting. Play meetings also provide a good opportunity for caregivers to socialize and find support; thus it is recommended that caregivers participate with their children as often as they can.

Caregivers can also participate in the professionally facilitated play sessions. The typical protocol of a 50-minute play session includes caregivers participating with their child in the second half of the session. This process is further described in the following section: 10 session guide for in-clinic AutPlay play groups. It is possible to facilitate AutPlay play groups without any parent participation, but this participation helps caregivers to better understand their child, improve their relationship with their child, and position them to be change agents in helping their child with their therapy needs.

Group Goals: AutPlay play groups always have basic goals and can include additional goals created by the therapist. The always goals include increasing the parent and child relationship, teaching parents how to have play time with their child, increasing the child's connection and engagement, increasing social comfort and experience for the child, and increasing parent support. The professional may design a group to include additional goals or may have some additional goals for certain children participating in the group.

The following guide presents a protocol for navigating ten play group sessions. AutPlay play groups follow a nondirective formally and consistent protocol from session to session. There is little variation from session one to session ten. The therapist does have the freedom to adjust and shift the group in ways that may be more effective for the group members. There should be a continuous reflective process to ensure the process is productive.

10 Session Guide for in Clinic Autplay Play Groups

Play Group Session One

Note: Professionals should review the step-by-step guide for beginning an AutPlay play group. This is located in the Appendix section of this book.

Length: Based on a 50-minute group session.

About This Week's Group: The professional should take note of any specific information they want to cover or address in this group session. The professional should review and prep for the session time. Are there any specific toys or materials that need to be highlighted? Does the room need any adjustments? Is the Session Overview Form for caregivers completed and ready to give to caregivers? During the first session, the children will follow the professional out of the waiting room and into the playroom. Caregivers will remain in the waiting room until they join the group with about 20 minutes left.

The Table: This is typically a literal table (usually a small child's table with chairs) but could also be a space on the floor, perhaps a blanket put down on the floor. This is for displaying selected toys or materials designed to promote social and play interaction. In AutPlay Play Groups, the children are free to roam the playroom or play space and play with anything they want, but sometimes the professional may want to place specific toys or materials on the "Table" to promote children playing together. Utilizing the "Table" concept is optional and may not be done in each session but should be considered as another tool to help promote engagement play.

Structuring Statement: Once the professional has greeted everyone in the waiting room and all the children are in the playroom, the therapist will make a simple structuring statement: "This is the playroom and you can play with anything you want in here and I (we) will be in here with you." Nothing else needs to be said or explained to the children at this time.

Play and Social Time: The children will have 35 minutes of nondirective play time. They may play with anything they want, and the professional(s) will move around the playroom making tracking and reflective statements and trying to encourage interactive play with themselves and other children in the group. The therapist is not aggressive and does not force any child to interact or play with anyone else. The professional makes consistent attempts and encourages but allows the process to develop at the child's comfort level. A reminder that play does not have to look one certain way; children can play the way that is meaningful to them. The professional is not teaching a way to play but rather attempting to join the child in their play.

Caregiver and Child Play Time: Caregivers join the group for the last 20 minutes. One of the professionals will get the caregivers from the waiting room when there are about 20 minutes left of the group time. Once the caregivers are in the playroom, they are given the following directive: "This is your time to play and interact with your child or any other parent and child and we will be in here with you." This is an opportunity for the therapist to further observe the caregiver/child interaction, and role model play attempts with the child and allow for more social play experiences. The professional will continue to track, reflect, and engage with any caregiver and/or child as opportunities arise.

Five-Minute Warning: When there are around five minutes left of the group time, the professional will make the following statement: "We have five minutes left of our group time today, then it will be time to go." The therapist makes another statement when there is one minute left of group time – "We have one-minute left of our group time and then it will be time to go." Parent and child are free to clean up any toys or materials or leave them. They are not asked or required to clean up after the group time is over.

Give Form to Caregivers: As the caregiver and child leave the playroom, the professional should give each caregiver the Session Overview Form. This form should have been completed by the professional prior to the group meeting. It provides the parents with information about what was addressed in the group meeting and information about the next week's caregiver-hosted play meeting.

Goodbye Ritual: Establishing a goodbye ritual is optional in AutPlay Play Groups, but professionals may want to consider the process. The goodbye ritual should be simple, and the same one should be used to end each group meeting. This could be as simple as giving a high five to each child and caregiver as they leave the playroom or waving and saying "bye" to each child as they leave the room. The professional can create their own unique goodbye ritual but should remember to keep it simple and be consistent in using the same process at the end of each group meeting.

Reflection: The therapist should plan time to reflect on the play group and each child in the group. The professional will want to take note of how each child participated in the group, if there were any signs of dysregulation, and how engagement and connection manifested. The professional will also assess if the group process seemed to work well for all group members or if adjustments need to be made.

Play Group Session Two

Length: Based on a 50-minute group session.

About This Week's Group: The professional should take note of any specific information they want to cover or address in this group session. The therapist should review and prepare for the session time. Are there any specific toys or materials that need to be highlighted? Does the room need any adjustments? Is the Session Overview Form for parents completed and ready to give to caregivers? Remember that caregivers will remain in the waiting room until they join the group with about 20 minutes left.

The Table: Utilizing the "Table" concept is optional and may not be done in each session but should be considered as another tool to help promote engagement and play. Possible toys for the table in session two might be Duplo Legos and/or building blocks.

Structuring Statement: The professional begins the group with a simple structuring statement – "This is the playroom and you can play with anything you want in here and I (we) will be in here with you." Nothing else needs to be said or explained to the children at this time.

Play and Social Time: The children will have 35 minutes of nondirective play time. They may play with anything they want, and the professional(s) will move around the playroom making tracking and reflective statements and trying to encourage interactive play with themselves and other children in the group. A reminder that tracking and reflective statements resemble those in child-centered play therapy (Landreth, 1991). A tracking statement is tracking what the child is doing, such as "You are scooping sand into the bucket" or "You are finished with the blocks and now you're playing with the cash register." Reflective statements reflect any emotion the child verbalizes or displays, such as "You are frustrated you can't get that lid off," "You like putting your hands in the sand," or "That makes you mad." The professional should try to make tracking and reflective statements periodically for each of the children in the group.

Caregiver and Child Play Time: Parents join the group for the last 20 minutes. Once the caregivers are in the playroom, they are given the following directive: "This is your time to play and interact with your child or any other caregiver and child and we will be in here with you." This is an opportunity for the professional to further observe the caregiver/child interaction, and role model play attempts with the child and allow for more social play experiences. The therapist can roam around the playroom and attempt to get involved with any of the caregivers and children's play time. The professional may even want to role model or help some caregivers as they attempt to play with their children. The professional can also encourage group play among the caregivers and children.

Five-Minute Warning: When there are around five minutes left of the group time, the professional will make the following statement: "We have five minutes left of our group time today, then it will be time to go." The therapist makes another statement when there is one minute left of group time – "We have one-minute left of our group time and then it will be time to go." Caregivers and children are free to clean up any toys or materials or leave them. They are not asked or required to clean up after the group time is over.

Give Form to Parents: As the parent and child leave the playroom, the professional should give each caregiver the Session Overview Form. This form should have been completed by the professional prior to the group meeting. It provides the caregivers with information about what was addressed in the group meeting and information about the next week's caregiver-hosted play meeting.

Goodbye Ritual: If a goodbye ritual was created and started in session one, it should be continued in session two. If one was not started in session one, it can be started in session two. Remember to keep the goodbye ritual simple and consistent. An example might be to have each child line up at the door, and as each child leaves, the professional gives them a fist pump. Another example would be as each child leaves the room, the child and professional do a quick goodbye dance move.

Reflection: The professional should plan time to reflect on the play group and each child in the group. The therapist will want to take note of how each child participated in the group if there were any signs of dysregulation, and how engagement and connection manifested. The professional will also assess if the group process seemed to work well for all group members or if adjustments need to be made.

Play Group Session Three

Length: Based on a 50-minute group session.

About This Week's Group: The therapist should take note of any specific information they want to cover or address in this group session. The professional should review and prep for the session time. Are there any specific toys or materials that need to be highlighted? Does the room need any adjustments? Is the Session Overview Form for caregivers completed and ready to give to caregivers?

The Table: Utilizing the "Table" concept is optional and may not be done in each session but should be considered as another tool to help promote engagement and play. Possible toys for the table in session three might be a couple of puzzles to put together (puzzles appropriate for the age and interests of the group members).

Structuring Statement: The professional begins the group with a simple structuring statement – "This is the playroom and you can play with anything you want in here and I (we) will be in here with you." Nothing else needs to be said or explained to the children at this time.

Play and Social Time: The children will have 35 minutes of nondirective play time. They may play with anything they want, and the professional(s) will move around the playroom making tracking and reflective statements and trying to encourage interactive play with themselves and other children in the group. Encouraging interactive play resembles the process of the FMA in AutPlay Therapy (Grant, 2017). The therapist periodically tries to get involved with what the child is playing. For example, if the child is playing in the sandtray, the professional will move beside the child and try to participate with the child and encourage interactive or reciprocal play. In AutPlay play groups, the professional can also try to involve other children in reciprocal play. The therapist should attempt to engage with each child in the group periodically but not force interactive play. A reminder that play does not have to look one certain way; children can play the way that is meaningful to them. The professional is not teaching a way to play but rather attempting to join the child in their play.

Caregiver and Child Play Time: Caregivers join the group for the last 20 minutes. Once the caregivers are in the playroom, they are given the following directive: "This is your time to play and interact with your child or any other caregiver and child and we will be in here with you." This is an opportunity for the professional to further observe the caregiver/child interaction, role model play attempts with the child, and allow for more connection and play experiences. It is likely that caregivers may have questions for the professional during this time. This is appropriate to a minimal degree and as questions relate directly to play times with their child or something happening in the moment. Other questions should be addressed at different times so the caregiver and child play time can be exclusively focused on the caregivers playing with or attempting to play with their child.

Five-Minute Warning: When there is around five minutes left of the group time, the professional will make the following statement: "We have five minutes left of our group time today, then it will be time to go." The professional makes another statement when there is one minute left of group time: "We have one-minute left of our group time and then it will be time to go." Parents and children are free to clean up any toys or materials or leave them. They are not asked or required to clean up after the group time is over.

Give Form to Parents: Give each caregiver the completed Session Overview Form as they leave the playroom.

Goodbye Ritual: If a goodbye ritual has been established, it should be implemented. Remember, the same goodbye ritual should be used to end each group meeting.

Reflection: The therapist should plan time to reflect on the play group and each child in the group. The professional will want to take note of how each child participated in the group if there were any signs of dysregulation, and how engagement and connection manifested. The professional will also assess if the group process seemed to work well for all group members or if adjustments need to be made. If parents express questions that cannot be answered during the play group, the professional should schedule a time to talk with caregivers.

Play Group Session Four

Length: Based on a 50-minute group session.

About This Week's Group: The professional should take note of any specific information they want to cover or address in this group session. The professional should review and prep for the session time. Are there any specific toys or materials that need to be highlighted? Does the room need any adjustments? Is the Session Overview Form for caregivers completed and ready to give to parents?

The Table: Utilizing the "Table" concept is optional and may not be done in each session but should be considered as another tool to help promote social play. Possible toys for the table in session four might be a large piece of white paper and crayons or markers.

Structuring Statement: The professional begins the group with a simple structuring statement: "This is the playroom and you can play with anything you want in here and I (we) will be in here with you." Nothing else needs to be said or explained to the children at this time.

Play and Social Time: The children will have 35 minutes of nondirective play time. They may play with anything they want, and the professional(s) will move around the playroom making tracking and reflective statements and trying to encourage interactive play with themselves and other children in the group.

Caregiver and Child Play Time: Parents join the group for the last 20 minutes. Once the caregivers are in the playroom, they are given the following directive: "This is your time to play and interact with your child or any other caregiver and child and we will be in here with you." This is an opportunity for the therapist to further observe the caregiver/child interaction, and role model play attempts with the child and allow for more social play experiences. The professional should continue to support each caregiver and child in their playtime. Some caregivers may struggle with engaging with their child. The therapist should be encouraging and supportive and assist any caregivers who may need help.

Five-Minute Warning: When there are around five minutes left of the group time, the professional will make the following statement: "We have five minutes left of our group time today, then it will be time to go." The professional makes another statement when there is one minute left of group time: "We have one-minute left of our group time and then it will be time to go." Caregivers and children are free to clean up any toys or materials or leave them. They are not asked or required to clean up after the group time is over.

Give Form to Caregivers: Give each parent the completed Session Overview Form as they leave the playroom.

Goodbye Ritual: If a goodbye ritual has been established, it should be implemented. Remember, the same goodbye ritual should be used to end each group meeting.

Reflection: The professional should plan time to reflect on the play group and each child in the group. The professional will want to take note of how each child participated in the group if there were any signs of dysregulation, and how engagement and connection manifested. The professional will also assess if the group process seemed to work well for all group members or if adjustments need to be made. If caregivers express questions that cannot be answered during the play group, the professional should schedule a time to talk with caregivers.

Play Group Session Five

Length: Based on a 50-minute group session.

About This Week's Group: The therapist should take note of any specific information they want to cover or address in this group session. The professional should review and prep for the session time. Are there any specific toys or materials that need to be highlighted? Does the room need any adjustments? Is the Session Overview Form for parents completed and ready to give to parents? At this point, about half of the group process has been completed. Professionals might consider having a short meeting with caregivers to evaluate how the process has been going for them. This meeting could be part of the group time or scheduled for a different time.

The Table: Utilizing the "Table" concept is optional and may not be done in each session but should be considered as another tool to help promote engagement and play. Possible toys for the table in session five might be a train track or race car track.

Structuring Statement: The professional begins the group with a simple structuring statement: "This is the playroom and you can play with anything you want in here and I (we) will be in here with you." Nothing else needs to be said or explained to the children at this time.

Play and Social Time: The children will have 35 minutes of nondirective play time. They may play with anything they want, and the professional(s) will move around the playroom making tracking and reflective statements and trying to encourage interactive play with themselves and other children in the group. This group meeting would be the halfway point in completing the group. The therapist should take note of any progress made toward interactive play and continue to encourage this with the group members. For those children who have started to play more socially and reciprocally, the professional will want to encourage this play to continue with other children. The professional may want to focus more of their engagement play efforts on those children who seem to present the most anxious and unsure.

Caregiver and Child Play Time: Parents join the group for the last 20 minutes. Once the caregivers are in the playroom, they are given the following directive: "This is your time to play and interact with your child or any other caregiver and child and we will be in here with you." This is the half-way portion of the group meetings. The professional should take note of the caregiver and child interactions and play of each member in the group and assess progress. Moving forward, the professional should focus more on those caregivers and children who are continuing to struggle with having play time.

Five-Minute Warning: When there are around five minutes left of the group time, the professional will make the following statement: "We have five minutes left of our group time today, then it will be time to go." The professional makes another statement when there is one minute left of group time: "We have one-minute left of our group time and then it will be time to go." Parents and children are free to clean up any toys or materials or leave them. They are not asked or required to clean up after the group time is over.

Give Form to Parents: Give each caregiver the completed Session Overview Form as they leave the playroom.

Goodbye Ritual: If a goodbye ritual has been established, it should be implemented. Remember, the same goodbye ritual should be used to end each group meeting.

Reflection: The therapist should plan time to reflect on the play group and each child in the group. The professional will want to take note of how each child participated in the group if there were any signs of dysregulation, and how engagement and connection manifested. The professional will also assess if the group process seemed to work well for all group members or if adjustments need to be made. If caregivers express questions that cannot be answered during the play group, the professional should schedule a time to talk with caregivers.

Play Group Session Six

Length: Based on a 50-minute group session.

About This Week's Group: The professional should take note of any specific information they want to cover or address in this group session. The professional should review and prep for the session time. Are there any specific toys or materials that need to be highlighted? Does the room need any adjustments? Is the

Session Overview Form for parents completed and ready to give to parents? At this point, the therapist will want to critically evaluate the children in the group in terms of how their engagement and play seem to be increasing and how their play time with their parents is progressing. The professional may want to target play interaction more specifically in encouraging social connection and play.

The Table: Utilizing the "Table" concept is optional and may not be done in each session but should be considered as another tool to help promote social play. Possible toys for the table in session six might be Mr. and Ms. Potato Head.

Structuring Statement: The professional begins the group with a simple structuring statement: "This is the playroom and you can play with anything you want in here and I (we) will be in here with you." Nothing else needs to be said or explained to the children at this time.

Play and Social Time: The children will have 35 minutes of nondirective play time. They may play with anything they want, and the professional(s) will move around the playroom making tracking and reflective statements and trying to encourage interactive play with themselves and other children in the group. Interactive play attempts should be focused on the children who seem to be struggling the most with engagement and connection. A reminder that play does not have to look one certain way; children can play the way that is meaningful to them. The therapist is not teaching a way to play but rather attempting to join the child in their play.

Caregiver and Child Play Time: Caregivers join the group for the last 20 minutes. Once the parents are in the playroom, they are given the following directive: "This is your time to play and interact with your child or any other caregiver and child and we will be in here with you." This is an opportunity for the professional to assist caregivers in having a positive and interactive play time with their child.

Five-Minute Warning: When there are around five minutes left of the group time, the professional will make the following statement: "We have five minutes left of our group time today, then it will be time to go." The therapist makes another statement when there is one minute left of group time: "We have one-minute left of our group time and then it will be time to go." Caregivers and children are free to clean up any toys or materials or leave them. They are not asked or required to clean up after the group time is over.

Give Form to Caregivers: Give each caregiver the completed Session Overview Form as they leave the playroom.

Goodbye Ritual: If a goodbye ritual has been established, it should be implemented. Remember, the same goodbye ritual should be used to end each group meeting.

Reflection: The professional should plan time to reflect on the play group and each child in the group. The professional will want to take note of how each child participated in the group, if there were any signs of dysregulation, and how engagement and connection manifested. The professional will also assess if the group process seemed to work well for all group members or if adjustments need to be made. If parents express questions that cannot be answered during the play group, the professional should schedule a time to talk with caregivers.

Play Group Session Seven

Length: Based on a 50-minute group session.

About This Week's Group: The professional should take note of any specific information they want to cover or address in this group session. The professional should review and prep for the session time. Are there any specific toys or materials that need to be highlighted? Does the room need any adjustments? Is the Session Overview Form for parents completed and ready to give to parents?

The Table: Utilizing the "Table" concept is optional and may not be done in each session but should be considered as another tool to help promote social play. Possible toys for the table in session seven might be a few board games or card games (age appropriate and aligns with group member interests).

Structuring Statement: The therapist begins the group with a simple structuring statement: "This is the playroom and you can play with anything you want in here and I (we) will be in here with you." Nothing else needs to be said or explained to the children at this time.

Play and Social Time: The children will have 35 minutes of nondirective play time. They may play with anything they want, and the professional(s) will move around the playroom making tracking and reflective statements and trying to encourage interactive play with themselves and other children in the group. Interactive play attempts should be focused on the children who seem the most unsure about engaging and connecting.

Caregiver and Child Play Time: Parents join the group for the last 20 minutes. Once the caregivers are in the playroom, they are given the following directive "This is your time to play and interact with your child or any other caregiver and child and we will be in here with you." This is an opportunity for the professional to assist caregivers in having a positive and interactive play time with their child.

Five-Minute Warning: When there are around five minutes left of the group time, the professional will make the following statement: "We have five minutes left of our group time today, then it will be time to go." The professional makes another statement when there is one minute left of group time: "We have one-minute left of our group time and then it will be time to go." Parents and children are free to clean up any toys or materials or leave them. They are not asked or required to clean up after the group time is over.

Give Form to Caregivers: Give each caregiver the completed Session Overview Form as they leave the playroom.

Goodbye Ritual: If a goodbye ritual has been established, it should be implemented. Remember, the same goodbye ritual should be used to end each group meeting.

Reflection: The professional should plan time to reflect on the play group and each child in the group. The therapist will want to take note of how each child participated in the group if there were any signs of dysregulation and how engagement and connection manifested. The professional will also assess if the group process seemed to work well for all group members or if adjustments need to be made. If caregivers express questions that cannot be answered during the play group, the professional should schedule a time to talk with caregivers.

Play Group Session Eight

Length: Based on a 50-minute group session.

About This Week's Group: The professional should take note of any specific information they want to cover or address in this group session. The professional should review and prep for the session time. Are there any specific toys or materials that need to be highlighted? Does the room need any adjustments? Is the Session Overview Form for parents completed and ready to give to parents?

The Table: Utilizing the "Table" concept is optional and may not be done in each session but should be considered as another tool to help promote social play. Possible toys for the table in session eight might be a bowling set or a ring toss game.

Structuring Statement: The professional begins the group with a simple structuring statement: "This is the playroom and you can play with anything you want in here and I (we) will be in here with you." Nothing else needs to be said or explained to the children at this time.

Play and Social Time: The children will have 35 minutes of nondirective play time. They may play with anything they want, and the professional(s) will move around the playroom making tracking and reflective statements and trying to encourage interactive play with themselves and other children in the group. Interactive play attempts should be focused on the children who seem the most anxious or unsure about engaging.

Caregiver and Child Play Time: Caregivers join the group for the last 20 minutes. Once the caregivers are in the playroom, they are given the following directive: "This is your time to play and interact with your child or any other parent and child and we will be in here with you." This is an opportunity for the professional to assist caregivers in having a positive and interactive play time with their child.

Five Minute Warning: When there are around five minutes left of the group time, the therapist will make the following statement: "We have five minutes left of our group time today, then it will be time to go." The professional makes another statement when there is one minute left of group time: "We have one-minute left of our group time and then it will be time to go." Caregivers and children are free to clean up any toys or materials or leave them. They are not asked or required to clean up after the group time is over.

Give Form to Caregivers: Give each parent the completed Session Overview Form as they leave the playroom.

Goodbye Ritual: If a goodbye ritual has been established, it should be implemented. Remember, the same goodbye ritual should be used to end each group meeting.

Reflection: The therapist should plan time to reflect on the play group and each child in the group. The professional will want to take note of how each child participated in the group if there were any signs of dysregulation and how engagement and connection manifested. The professional will also assess if the group process seemed to work well for all group members or if adjustments need to be made. If caregivers express questions that cannot be answered during the play group, the professional should schedule a time to talk with caregivers.

Play Group Session Nine

Length: Based on a 50-minute group session.

About This Week's Group: The therapist should take note of any specific information they want to cover or address in this group session. The professional should review and prep for the session time. Are there any specific toys or materials that need to be highlighted? Does the room need any adjustments? Is the Session Overview Form for caregivers completed and ready to give to parents?

The Table: Utilizing the "Table" concept is optional and may not be done in each session but should be considered as another tool to help promote engagement and play. Possible toys for the table in session nine might be puppets.

Structuring Statement: The professional begins the group with a simple structuring statement: "This is the playroom and you can play with anything you want in here and I (we) will be in here with you." Nothing else needs to be said or explained to the children at this time.

Play and Engagement Time: The children will have 35 minutes of nondirective play time. They may play with anything they want, and the professional(s) will move around the playroom making tracking and reflective statements and trying to encourage interactive play with themselves and other children in the group. Interactive play attempts should be focused on the children who are the most unsure and on encouraging children to engage with each other.

Caregiver and Child Play Time: Caregivers join the group for the last 20 minutes. Once the caregivers are in the playroom, they are given the following directive: "This is your time to play and interact with your child or any other caregiver and child and we will be in here with you." This is an opportunity for the professional to assist parents in having a positive and interactive play time with their child. The professional should note that there is only one group meeting left after this one. If the professional feels it is necessary, they could meet individually with any caregiver and child who may still be struggling and could benefit from a more focused session with the professional to work on engagement or caregiver/child play times.

Five-Minute Warning: When there are around five minutes left of the group time, the professional will make the following statement: "We have five minutes left of our group time today, then it will be time to go." The professional makes another statement when there is one minute left of group time: "We have one-minute left of our group time and then it will be time to go." Caregivers and children are free to clean up any toys or materials or leave them. They are not asked or required to clean up after the group time is over.

Give Form to Caregivers: Give each caregiver the completed Session Overview Form as they leave the playroom.

Goodbye Ritual: If a goodbye ritual has been established, it should be implemented. Remember, the same goodbye ritual should be used to end each group meeting.

Reflection: The therapist should plan time to reflect on the play group and each child in the group. The professional will want to take note of how each child participated in the group, if there were any signs of dysregulation, and how engagement and connection manifested. The therapist will also assess if the group process seemed to work well for all group members or if adjustments need to be made. If caregivers express questions that cannot be answered during the play group, the professional should schedule a time to talk with caregivers.

Play Group Session Ten

Length: Based on a 50-minute group session.

About This Week's Group: The professional should take note of any specific information they want to cover or address in this group session. The professional should review and prep for the session time. Are there any specific toys or materials that need to be highlighted? Does the room need any adjustments? Is the Session Overview Form for caregivers completed and ready to give to caregivers? This is the final in-clinic group meeting. The therapist may want to have a short meeting with caregivers to discuss participation in future groups or possibly continue with the play group. AutPlay Play Groups can be ongoing, and this is often encouraged as neurodivergent children typically benefit from more than ten sessions.

The Table: Utilizing the "Table" concept is optional and may not be done in each session but should be considered as another tool to help promote engagement and social play. Possible toys for the table in session ten might be a sandtray and sandtray toys.

Structuring Statement: The professional begins the group with a simple structuring statement: "This is the playroom and you can play with anything you want in here and I (we) will be in here with you." The therapist should mention to the children that this will be the last group meeting.

Play and Engagement Time: This is the last play group meeting, and the professional should continue with the same process as they have been implementing. The play time length might be shortened to around 25 minutes to provide more time for a final goodbye ritual and any closure processes that need to be implemented. The children will continue to play with anything they want, and the professional(s) will move around the playroom, making tracking and reflective statements and trying to encourage interactive play with themselves and other children in the group. Interactive play attempts should be focused on the children who seem the most unsure.

Caregiver and Child Play Time: This is the last session, and the caregiver and child play time proceeds as usual with the parents joining the group for the last 20 minutes. The professional may want to shorten the caregiver and child play time to have more time for the final goodbye ritual and to discuss any closure issues with the caregivers. This would also be an appropriate time to discuss moving forward with continuing the group, starting a new group, or working individually with some of the parents and children.

Five-Minute Warning: When there are around five minutes left of the group time, the professional will make the following statement "We have five minutes left of our group time today, then it will be time to go." The professional makes another statement when there is one minute left of group time: "We have one-minute left of our group time and then it will be time to go." Caregivers and children are free to clean up any toys or materials or leave them. They are not asked or required to clean up after the group time is over.

Give Form to Caregivers: Give each parent the completed Session Overview Form as they leave the playroom. This is the last session, and this should be noted on the form. There is technically one more caregiver-hosted play meeting scheduled for the next week; this should be noted on the form. Caregivers are encouraged to continue to have play meetings with the other children and caregivers as they wish.

Goodbye Ritual: Since this is the last group session. The professional may want to take more time and express a goodbye and thank you for playing in the group to the children and allow them to express a goodbye to the other children if they would like. The therapist should have prepared and given to each caregiver and child a certificate of completion. A sample certificate of completion is provided in the appendix section of this book. If it has been established that the group will continue to meet, then the standard goodbye ritual can be implemented.

Reflection: The professional may want to write a final note to caregivers. The note can highlight goals worked on and achieved through the group, progress that was made, suggestions for further therapy, encouragement to continue to have play times with their child at home, and encouragement to continue to meet with other children and caregivers for "play dates."

References

Axline, V. M. (1969). *Play therapy*. Ballantine Books.

Grant, R. J. (2023). *The AutPlay therapy handbook: Integrative family play therapy with neurodivergent children*. Routledge.

Hogeveen, J., & Grafman, J. (2021). Alexithymia. *Handbook of clinical neurology, 183*, 47–62. https://doi.org/10.1016/B978-0-12-822290-4.00004-9

Knell, S. M. (1997). *Cognitive behavioral play therapy*. Rowman & Littlefield.

Landreth, G. L. (1991). *Play therapy: The art of the relationship*. Accelerated Development.

Ray, D. C., Sullivan, J. M., & Carlson, S. E. (2012). Relational intervention: Child-centered play therapy with children on the autism spectrum. In L. Gallo-Lopez & L. C. Rubin (Eds.), *Play-based interventions for children and adolescents with autism spectrum disorders* (pp. 159–175). Routledge/Taylor & Francis Group.

Sweeney, D. S., Baggerly, J. N., & Ray, D. C. (2014). *Group play therapy: A dynamic approach*. Routledge.

Chapter 7

AutPlay® Therapy Social Groups with Older Children and Adolescents (10 Session Framework)

Social-Focused Groups

Social navigation groups are an intervention strategy in which two or more neurodivergent children come together and discover individual and group relational and social dynamics. The members can share what they believe their social strengths and challenges are, and caregivers can also help articulate what they have noticed. Group members can relationally work through specific social navigation needs with the support of the professional. These groups have been found to be effective in navigating many possible social needs, including social interaction, perspective-taking, handling disagreements, advocating, and managing emotions. There are many potential benefits for implementing social navigation groups for neurodivergent children; these benefits include possible increased relational learning by placing peers in closer proximity to each other and increasing the likelihood of generalization and peer satisfaction outside the social navigation group.

AutPlay social groups are based off the AutPlay Therapy structured intervention phase of therapy. In this phase of therapy, the therapist is assessing the best-fitting therapy approach for the child and their identified needs. One possible option is to have the child and caregiver both present during the sessions and teach directive play therapy interventions, which are practiced during session times. The therapist teaches the parent how to continue to implement the interventions at home between sessions. This process continues until therapy goals are met. AutPlay Therapy directive play therapy interventions are specifically designed to meet a child where they are in terms of their age and developmental needs. AutPlay Therapy directive play therapy interventions are designed to help increase social navigation and other needs such as emotional regulation, anxiety reduction, and relationship development. The AutPlay Therapy Framework considers the possible challenge social navigation that may be present in neurodivergent children without ever broadly assuming particular "abilities" should or need to be implemented. The professional values the neurodivergent way to play when implementing directive play interventions so that neurodivergent children can participate and feel more confident in the play engagement.

DOI: 10.4324/9781003468370-8

AutPlay social navigation groups mimic the structured intervention phase in AutPlay Therapy in many ways. In each clinic meeting, the group participants are taught a specific play technique, one in which the group has reported having a play preference or interest. The play interventions are also selected to focus on improving identified group goals. Caregivers are then encouraged to support the interventions being addressed at home between group meetings. Parents are taught how to host a "hang out time" or meeting with the group participants outside of the clinical setting. This is an opportunity for the participants to have a less formal gathering to practice being with each other. Incorporating caregiver involvement and the utilization of directive play therapy interventions are both processes in AutPlay social navigation groups taken directly from the AutPlay Therapy Framework.

It is also possible to implement AutPlay social groups from a nondirective perspective. In this version, directive play interventions would not be used, and the therapist would provide less structure for the meetings. The participants would come together and lead the social navigation of the group. This would be a time where the members could be with each other and interact as they like and at their comfort level. The therapist might provide accessible items and materials that the group members have expressed that they like, such as Lego bricks, art supplies, video games, etc. The members could freely play and interact with each other, and the professional would provide tracking and reflective statements and general facilitation but primarily let the children navigate as they liked. This version of AutPlay social groups focuses more on social connection and nondivertive play therapy philosophy in contrast with groups that have directive interventions designed to address identified group therapy goals. Both types of groups can be beneficial. For the purpose of this chapter, we will focus primarily on directive play intervention groups.

Pragmatics of AutPlay Therapy Social Groups

Definition of AutPlay Therapy Social Groups: These groups focus on providing social experience and are designed for elementary, middle, and high school-aged children who are neurodivergent or could benefit from positive relational social group work. Children and adolescents who are neurotypical or if their neurodivergence is unsure can also participate. The support needs of the child do not matter, but they must be able to participate on some level in structure and/or directive play interventions; otherwise, participating in an AutPlay play group would be more appropriate.

Role of the Professional: The professional organizes and facilitates the AutPlay social group process. The therapist is a player and an encourager for both the children and the caregivers. Often, the professional also serves as a role model and instructor. The professional is active in the social groups by teaching specific social play interventions, establishing limits when necessary, and providing support and strategies to caregivers.

Structure: AutPlay social groups are typically 20 group sessions each lasting around one hour. The group begins with a meeting in the professional's clinic where group goals are taught and practiced through various play therapy interventions. The next week, the group participants meet outside of the clinic to have a less formal "hang out" time. This meeting is hosted by one of the participants' caregivers. The meetings alternate in this fashion week to week for 20 meetings – ten in clinic group sessions and ten outside "hang out" meetings. A step-by-step organization and structure guide for starting an AutPlay social group is provided in the appendix section of this book.

Generating Interest in a Group: Professionals should assess in their local community the need for social groups. This can be done by contacting local agencies that work with neurodivergent children and adolescents, contacting school programs, and checking with local caregiver support groups.

Organization of a Group: The therapist should decide on a possible start date and location for the group. The professional should also prepare any forms needed for the group and begin to market the group. A sample marketing flier is provided in the appendix section of this book.

Assessing/Screening Group Members: It is important that group members are as similar as possible when it comes to age, developmental level, and support needs. Gender tends to not be as important as having children in the same group who may have similar interests and/or social needs. When you have groups with many ages and several different levels of support, you lose some of the environmental conditions that help develop social group satisfaction. The Intake Form and Group Readiness Questionnaire found in the appendix section of this book can be used to help assess group participants.

The professional should meet with each caregiver and child who might be interested in participating in a social group. This meeting is an opportunity to complete necessary paperwork, assess the child's strengths and needs level, and decide if the child would be an appropriate fit for the group that is beginning. If the child is assessed to not be ready for a group experience, the therapist should try to offer a meeting with the child for individual therapy and working toward joining a group. The professional can offer more than one group. This might be especially helpful if there are different ages and support need levels wanting to attend; the professional could offer multiple groups, matching the children with the best-fitting group. It might be necessary to place some children on a group wait list until there are enough children interested in participating in a group that are at the same age and need level.

Who Can Participate: Any child or adolescent can participate in an AutPlay social group. Participants do not need a formal neurodivergent category diagnosis. Although a primary focus of the group is neurodivergent needs, any child who might benefit from the social navigation work of the group could participate.

Group Size: The typical size of a group should be four to six children, with no more than eight. Anything larger will negatively affect the ability of the group to naturally connect and work on social navigation. Groups can be smaller and still be beneficial, but larger groups should be avoided. It would likely be better to have two groups of four than one group of eight. The minimum number of participants for a group is two. Therapists should strive for a ratio of one adult for every two children, so the larger the group size, the more adults that will be needed to facilitate the group. These are recommendations for group size. This will vary depending on the age and possible connection difficulties of the participants. It might be possible for one professional to work with a group of four children if they were older children and they had many similarities in interests and strengths/needs.

Length of Group Meetings: The length of time a group meets may vary depending on the professional's preference, but the group structure for AutPlay social groups is based on a one-hour group session. Some therapists may prefer to lengthen the group time.

Number of Group Meetings: AutPlay social groups meet for ten in-clinic formal teaching times and ten outside of the clinic less formal "hang out" times. There are a total of 20 meetings. The formal and informal meetings alternate from week to week. The first week the group meets in the clinic; and the next week they meet outside of the clinic. The professional does not attend the outside-of-the-clinic meeting; this is hosted by one of the participant's caregivers. The therapist can begin new groups at any time or start another group when one ends, and the new groups can include some of the same participants from a previous group. It is important to formally end a group after the 20 meetings to give children a clean opportunity to leave the group.

Play Development: Since much of the group focus will be on participating in play therapy interventions, it is important to assess each child's play preferences and interests. The AutPlay Groups Assessment of Play Form is provided in the appendix section of this book. The professional will give the caregiver the play assessment to complete as part of the group intake process prior to the group beginning.

Social Navigation Development: AutPlay social groups provide an integrative process of clinical and natural opportunity for children and adolescents to develop positive relational and social satisfaction. A formal, more directive play intervention process happens during the in-clinic meetings, while a less formal, more naturalist process happens outside of the clinic meetings. Both experiences are important for participants to feel invested and accepted.

Group Meeting Locations: The professional will likely have in-clinic meetings at their clinic or some arranged meeting place. It is ideal for the in-clinic meeting location to stay consistent throughout the duration of the group. For the caregiver hosted, outside the clinic meetings, there are many options where a group could meet (this is typically decided on by the parent who is hosting). A common setting such as a caregiver's home, a church, or a support group meeting facility would certainly work. It is highly encouraged that some of the

Table 7.1 Meeting Places for Parent Hosted Social Groups

Arcade	Nature Center
Botanical Garden	Area Lake
Special Events (Art Fest, Cider Days, Autism Fairs)	Zoo
YMCA/Community Center	Public Pool
Discovery Center	Various Stores
Restaurants	Movie Theater
Incredible Pizza	Jump House
Sporting Event	Museum
Farms	Fair/Carnival/Circus
Amusement Park	Miniature Golf
Go Carts	Fishing/Canoeing/Hiking
Picnic	Public Library
Pottery Studio	Farmers Market
State Parks	Imax
Ice Skating Rink/Roller Skating	Road Trip
Neighborhood Walk	Mall
Church Events	Grocery Store
Pumpkin Patch	Post Office
Horse Stables	Animal Shelter

social group meetings occur in public. This may be a certain event or specific activity designed for children; it may simply be going to a restaurant or park. Some parents may need help in deciding where to meet. Table 7.1 provides some meeting place options for caregivers. Also, the professional should communicate to parents that the caregiver-hosted meetings should not include any formal social navigation interventions. This is a time for the participants to be together and practice natural socialization. The caregivers can help their child to interact and provide encouragement, but there should be no pressure or purposeful teaching. The participants need this time to be with other children and enjoy a group experience.

It is helpful for parents to understand the dynamics of the children in the group and where each child is in terms of social confidence and tolerance for certain situations, such as any sensory issues or fears related to certain environments. Any information about any of the group participants that would guide the selection of a location or event for a caregiver-hosted meeting should be shared with the caregivers to avoid any potential issues. Where to meet and the type of hangout experience should be decided on and communicated the week before the parent-hosted meeting. Typically, the professional will have this information and share it with all the children and caregivers at the end of the in-clinic meeting. This information is included on the Session Overview Form (located in the appendix section) that is given to the parents at the end of each in-clinic meeting.

Handling Uncomfortable Behavior: The professional will want to choose one of the limit-setting models defined in this book and explain the limit-setting model to the participants during the first meeting. The therapist should use the limit-setting model consistently. Each model provides for a final decision of ending the group time for the child if they are having dysregulation difficulties that are affecting other group members. The professional should be patient and implement limits at a minimum. It is expected that there will be some unexpected and dysregulation behavior. If it is something the therapist can work with and modify easily, then there is no need for further limits. If possible, the professional should establish a break room or area that the participants can go to if they are needing a break. This is something the professional can lead the child to, or the child can initiate a break themselves. If a break room is established, the professional should explain this to the participants during the first session.

When parents are hosting a group meeting, the professional will not typically be present. The caregivers may need a brief instruction on how to handle dysregulating behavior during outside of clinic meetings. It's important to explain to caregivers that dysregulation will likely occur during a caregiver-hosted meeting. If a parent has certain strategies they typically implement to help their child calm, the caregiver should implement these strategies. If a caregiver feels like they need to leave the meeting, this is acceptable. The caregiver and child should leave, and they can try again at the next meeting. Other parents should get involved only if the caregiver of the child with significant dysregulation asks for assistance. It is important that the caregiver of the child with the dysregulation is the primary person addressing their child and trying to manage the behavior.

Caregivers as Co-Change Agents: Caregivers participate in the AutPlay social groups. In AutPlay Therapy, one of the ways caregivers work with the professional is in learning interventions to help their child progress toward therapy goals. In AutPlay social groups, parents host a group meeting outside of the clinic to help further the acquisition of relational and social gains. This process is fully explained to caregivers during the initial consultation about the social group. Any training, suggestions, or help a caregiver may need should be provided by the professional. If a parent has concerns and would like suggestions for hosting a group time, the therapist should meet with the caregiver and provide the information they are requesting. The professional should communicate to parents that they are an important part of the group process and empower caregivers to feel confident in their participation.

When parents host a group meeting, other caregivers should participate in each group meeting as much as possible. It may not be necessary for every caregiver to be at every meeting if caregivers are comfortable with others taking care of their children (this will depend on the size of the group and the interest level of group participants). It is important that there are enough parents at each group meeting to care for the children and facilitate the group. Social groups provide a good opportunity for caregivers to socialize and find support; thus, it is recommended that caregivers participate with their children as often as they can.

10 Session Guide for in Clinic Autplay Social Navigation Groups

Note: Professionals should review the step-by-step guide for beginning an AutPlay group. This is located in the Appendix section of this book.

Social Group Session One

Length: Based on a one-hour group session.

About This Week's Group: The professional should take note of any specific information they want to cover or address in this group session. The professional should review and prep for the session time. Are there any materials needed for the intervention? Does the therapist have an ice breaker and closing activity planned? Is the Session Overview Form for caregivers completed and ready to give to caregivers?

Welcome Ice Breaker: Welcome the participants and ask each participant to share their name and something they like doing. It can be a video game, a sport, or any activity. Each professional should go first, introducing themselves and role modeling how to share as well as what information to share. This ice breaker should be brief, only taking about ten minutes.

First Session Information: In the first session only, the therapist will briefly go over the structure of the group sessions, what the participants can expect each week, and how the caregiver hosted outside of the clinic meetings work. The professional will cover any group expectations, such as being positive with each other. The therapist will also want to cover the limit-setting model that will be used to address any limits that need to be set. If there is a process for participants to take a break if they are feeling dysregulated, this process should be explained to the group participants.

Anything to Share: This will be an active part of each group session where the participants will have an opportunity to share anything they would like with the group. In the first session, it is likely there will not be much sharing, but this may increase as the group meets more often. The anything to share time gives the group participants an opportunity to get to know each other better, practice sharing, become more comfortable, and engage in reciprocal conversation. Professionals should monitor for any limit setting that is needed, such as perspective taking, subject matter, and negative responses.

Implement the Play Intervention: A sample intervention for children (elementary age) and adolescents (middle and high school age) is provided. The professional is welcome to use the interventions in this book and implement them in any order that they feel is appropriate. The therapist can also use their own play interventions that they have created or acquired from other sources.

Process and Application of the Play Intervention: The professional will want to allow for some processing and application of the intervention. An example of processing and application is provided at the end of each intervention description.

Goodbye Ritual: The therapist should end each session with a goodbye ritual. This can change from session to session, or the professional can repeat the same goodbye ritual each time. An example would be creating a special group handshake that each participant does to each other as they leave the group. This should be brief, only taking about five minutes.

Give Form to Caregivers: As the children leave the group session, the professional should give each caregiver the Session Overview Form. Therapists will want to have the form completed prior to the group session.

Group Session One Example Play Intervention for Children

Activity: Quiet and Loud.
Target Area(s): Identity, self-worth, body awareness.
Level: Children.
Materials Needed: None.
Introduction: Neurodivergent children often have a different way of navigating. Other people may not always appreciate the child's neurotype, and the child may receive negative messages about themselves. This intervention uses body awareness to help children understand they are valuable and fine no matter who they are, how they feel, and what they do.

Instructions:

1   The professional tells the group that they are going to do some activities that help the group appreciate being themselves.
2   The professional first expresses that sometimes we may feel quiet and sometimes we may feel loud. We can feel however we feel, and this is okay. The professional demonstrates pressing their hands together in front of them and begins by saying this is our way of being quiet.
3   The professional and group practice saying things quietly and tip-toeing around the room. The professional explains that sometimes in some situations we may feel like being quiet, and this is okay.
4   The professional move their hands all the way apart and until both arms are fully stretched out. The professional explains this is our way of being loud.
5   The professional and group practice saying things loudly and stomping around the room. The professional explains that sometimes in some situations we may feel like being loud, and this is okay.
6   The professional can follow up on the activity by discussing times and situations where they have felt quiet or loud in their thoughts and body. The professional and group can also practice more examples of quiet and loud.

Processing and Application: This play intervention works on increasing awareness and acceptance of self. Body movement is utilized to better help the child connect to their understanding of their neurodivergent self. This intervention can be played multiple times to help the children progress in self-worth, especially related to their neurodivergence.

Group Session One Example Social Navigation Intervention for Adolescents

Activity: Divide and Conquer.
Target Area(s): Executive functioning, connection, engagement, and teamwork.
Level: Adolescents.
Materials Needed: Balloons.
Introduction: Neurodivergent adolescents may often have discomfort working with others and participating as part of a team. This intervention focuses on helping adolescents to notice others, work cooperatively, strategize to solve a problem and work with another person to accomplish a task. It incorporates a teamwork concept in a fun and engaging game format.

Instructions:

1 The professional explains to the group that they are going to play a game where the focus is on working together as a team to accomplish a task.
2 The professional divides the group into pairs, and each pair chooses an area to stand in the room.
3 The professional explains to the group that they can position themselves and their feet anywhere in the room, but once in place, they have to pretend that their feet are stuck to the floor and cannot be moved. They should strategize the best formation for keeping their balloon in the air.
4 The adolescent and their partner hit a balloon in the air back and forth and try to keep it from touching the ground without moving their feet.
5 The professional should spend some time discussing with the group the concept of working together and teamwork and that the only way to succeed at the game is by paying attention to each other and working as a team.
6 The professional should also encourage the group participants to strategize and develop a plan deciding where each person will stand to cover the most room space.
7 If the balloon hits the ground, the pair can decide on a different place to stand and start over, seeing if they can keep the balloon in the air longer. The game can be started over and played multiple times.

Processing and Application: The professional should process and ask the group what it felt like to work with another person, what felt easy, and what felt difficult. The professional can also ask participants to share about real life experiences where they had to work as part of a team or with another person to accomplish something. This intervention promotes executive functioning, cooperation, body awareness, personal space, and self-control. Participants must work together to keep the balloon from hitting the ground, communicate to coordinate where they are going to stand to try and cover as much space as possible in the room, and often readjust/strategize and discuss how they are going to keep the balloon from touching the ground.

Social Navigation Group Session Two

Length: Based on a one-hour group session.

About This Week's Group: The professional should continue to take note of any specific information they want to cover in this group session, as well as review and prep for the session. Prep would include having a list of statements ready for the icebreaker activity, having a general joy or sorrow ready to share, and finding a goodbye poem for the ending ritual. Materials for this session should be created and displayed. The ice breaker and closing activity should be practiced, and the Session Overview Form ready to give to caregivers.

Welcome Ice Breaker: *That's Like Me* icebreaker carries over from session one in which clients can share something about themselves. The therapist begins by stating something about themselves (example: "I love winter"). Any group member who agrees with this statement calls out 'That's Like Me'. Each group member can then share a statement about themselves, and other group members can state "That's Like Me" when they agree with the statement. The professional should be prepared to prompt members with ideas if needed (examples include favorite season, favorite food, worst school subject, members in family, etc.). The ice breaker should take five to ten minutes maximum.

Anything to Share: There may be more sharing during this group session, but there may also be some participants who are not ready. It may be helpful for the professional to ask the group members if they have any joys or sorrows to share from the past week and model an example if needed. The therapist should keep their joy or sorrow general so as not to influence any group member's responses (for example, "I had a great dinner last night," "I didn't have an umbrella on the rainy-day last Thursday," etc.). The professional is an active listener at this time and monitors for any limit setting needed.

Implement the Social Navigation Intervention: A sample intervention for children and adolescents is provided. The professional is welcome to use the social navigation interventions in this book and implement them in any order that they feel is appropriate. The therapist can also use their own social navigation interventions, which they have created or acquired from other sources.

Process and Application of the Intervention: The therapist will want to allow for some processing and application of the social navigation intervention. An example of processing and application is provided at the end of each social intervention description.

Goodbye Ritual: The professional should end the session with the goodbye ritual from the previous session or create a new one for this session. An example would be reading a poem found online about saying goodbye.

Give Form to Caregivers: As the children leave the group session, the professional should give each parent the Session Overview Form. The professional will want to have the form completed prior to the group session.

Group Session Two: Example Social Navigation Intervention for Children

Activity: Speak.
Target Area(s): Advocating, sharing with others.
Level: Children.
Materials Needed: One mouth template glued onto a craft stick and enough ear templates glued onto craft sticks for each member of the group (the professional can draw and cut out mouth and ear pics or print off templates online). Multicolor crayons, or multiple shades of peach, brown and black crayons, and a one-minute sand timer (can also use the timer on a cell phone, etc.).
Introduction: *Speak* is a fun way for children to practice speaking in a group and being comfortable speaking up for themselves. This can be difficult, so the professional wants to keep it light and encouraging. The ear and mouth templates are a fun way to remind the members what their role is as the speaker or the listener. The professional does not expect any group member to speak for the entire minute but encourages each child to attempt some verbalization and does set a limit of one-minute speaking. The professional is also not expecting a continued conversation on the same subject matter; that is an advanced communication that is not necessary for this activity. Children can speak about whatever they want during their time.

Instructions:

1 The professional tells the group that they are going to complete an activity that helps all of us learn how to speak about something they like.
2 The professional keeps the mouth prop and passes out one ear prop to each group member. Members are encouraged to color the ear if they like with the crayons provided.
3 The professional explains that in this game, whoever holds the mouth is the speaker. The speaker will turn over the sand timer and then talk about whatever they want for one minute. They can talk less than that, but not

more than one minute. Those who hold the ear props are the listeners. The ears need to listen to the speaker and not interrupt. It may be important to remind the listeners that we are only focusing on not interrupting. Many individuals can listen without eye contact, sitting still, etc., and we are not focusing on that.

4 The professional begins by holding the mouth prop up to their mouth and speaking for one minute. The group members hold the ear props up to one of their ears and listen.

5 When one minute is up, the professional congratulates the members on their hard work and may need to remind the members of expectations. The professional then passes the mouth to a group member and takes their ear prop. The activity is completed when every person has a turn as the speaker.

Processing and Application: The professional discusses with the group members the importance of using their voices to share with others and to advocate for their needs. The group discusses when this would be important at home, school, and other environments. The professional makes sure each group member has the mouth and ear templates to take home for practice.

Group Session Two: Example Social Navigation Intervention for Adolescents

Activity: Where I Stand.
Target Area(s): Sharing with others, socializing with others, and perspective-taking.
Level: Adolescents.
Materials Needed: One long piece of yarn taped to the floor (yarn should be long enough to have all group members stand comfortably on the yarn with space between them). Two index cards taped to the floor on each end of the yarn. The word "YES!" should be written on one index card; 'NO' on the other index card. A sample of yes and no questions is provided at the end of this activity description.
Introduction: Neurodivergent adolescents may have difficulties with understanding the different points of view of others (perspective taking). This intervention helps them notice that other peers may not think or feel the same way they do. This intervention also allows group members to share and socialize in a structured format.

Instructions:

1 Before the group members arrive, the professional tapes a long piece of yarn to the floor and places the yes index card at one end and the no index card at the other.

2 The professional explains to the group that they are going to play a game to get to know each other better. The professional explains that they will say out loud a statement, and each group member should respond to the statement by standing on the yarn to the degree of how they feel about the statement. The closer they are to the "YES!" index card, the more they agree with the statement; the closer they are to the 'NO!' index card, the more they disagree with the statement. (The professional may need to check for understanding and give a few examples.)

3 The professional says aloud the first statement and gives everyone time to choose where they are going to stand on the yarn. When everyone has chosen a place, the professional invites any group member to share why they chose where they stood on the line. The professional may also suggest that group members look around and notice how members feel differently about the question.

4 The professional continues this game until all statements are read.

Processing and Application: The professional is making sure during this activity that group members are being respectful of differing opinions. The group discusses what they learned about each other and themselves during the activity. Some questions the professional can ask include: Were you surprised about anything you learned? Were any of the statements difficult for you to decide where to stand? After listening to other group members, were you considering moving to a different spot on the yarn?

Sample Yes and No Questions

- I like to have people around me
- I sleep well at night
- I do well in school
- I am honest
- I do my homework
- I play computer games
- I am smart
- I am a happy person
- I eat healthy
- I have friends
- I help my siblings
- I have meltdowns
- I love to eat sweets
- I play outside
- I like to swim
- I live with my mom and dad
- I am funny

- I wake up easily in the morning
- My teacher likes me
- I do my own laundry
- I like to play sports
- Math is my best subject

Social Navigation Group Session Three

Length: Based on a one-hour group session.

About This Week's Group: The therapist should continue to take note of any specific information they want to cover in this group session, as well as review and prep for the session. Prep would include having examples of ways to line up for the icebreaker by having a general joy or sorrow ready to share and by having the word 'goodbye' in different languages. Materials for this session should be created and displayed. The ice breaker and closing activity should be practiced, and the Session Overview Form ready to give to caregivers.

Welcome Ice Breaker: *Line Up* is a short game that allows the group members to work together while discovering a bit more about each other. The professional calls out, "Everyone line up according to..." (examples include youngest to oldest, alphabetically older, shortest to tallest, etc.) Group members discover together how they all need to line up.

Anything to Share: The therapist should follow the same suggestions from group session one or two.

Implement the Social Navigation Intervention: The professional can use the interventions provided below, in the appendix of this book, or one of their own.

Process and Application of the Intervention: An example of processing and application is provided at the end of each social intervention description.

Goodbye Ritual: Teach the group members ways to say goodbye in other languages and have them choose one goodbye they will say to others.

Spanish:	Adios
French:	Au Revoir
German:	Auf Wiedersehen
Italian:	Arrivederci
Japanese:	Sayonara
Hindi:	Namaste
Arabic:	Ma'a as-salaama
Hawaiian:	Aloha

Give Form to Caregiver: As the children leave the group session, the professional should give each caregiver the Session Overview Form. The therapist will want to have the form completed prior to the group.

Group Session Three: Example Social Navigation Intervention for Children

Activity: Space Please!

Target Area: Identifying needs and social boundaries, understanding others' body language, understanding perspective-taking, and advocating for self.

Level: Children.

Materials Needed: Several pool noodles, some original size, some cut in half, thirds, and quarters.

Introduction: The *Space Please!* activity allows group members to determine how much personal space they need to feel comfortable. They will also discover others may need more or less personal space than they do. Often, neurodivergents may believe that their comfort level mirrors others, and this can cause difficulty with peer relationships. Since it can be very hard for all children to recognize the social cues of their peers, children may not understand they are standing too close or too far away from someone. This activity will help students realize they may need to ask their peers if they are comfortable with where they are standing or tell peers they need more space. The professional should also ensure the participants that if any distance feels too dysregulating, they have the right to opt out of the activity.

Instructions:

1 Divide the group into pairs. If there is an odd number, the professional should be a group member.
2 Give each pair a full-sized pool noodle. Instruct each group member to place one end of the noodle on each of their stomachs and hold it there.
3 Keeping the pool noodle on each of their bellies, pairs should have a conversation. If the group members struggle with this, the professional could ask a general question to stimulate conversation.
4 When finished, have pairs drop the full-sized noodle and give each group member a half-sized pool noodle. Follow the same directions as with the full-sized pool noodle.
5 When finished, have pairs drop the half-sized pool noodle and give each group member a third-sized, then a quarter-sized pool noodle. Follow the same directions as with the previous sized noodles.

Processing and Application: Once this activity has been completed, the group members should come together and sit in a circle with each other. The professional should ask each group member when they felt the most comfortable as far as personal space. Was one noodle-length too close, too far, just right? Point out after each participant shares the similarities and differences they shared. Discuss ways that group members could share with their caregivers, teachers, and peers the amount of personal space they need, as well as ways to decide if they are giving others enough personal space.

Group Session Three: Example Social Navigation Intervention for Adolescents

Activity: Personal Space.
Target Area(s): Identifying needs and social boundaries, understanding others' body language, understanding perspective-taking, and advocating for self.
Level: Adolescents.
Materials Needed: Several balls of yarn and scissors.
Introduction: This is an excellent way for clients to work on recognizing the body language and facial expressions of their peers and how to advocate for their own needs. It can also help them see that everyone has different needs and that personal space is personal to all. All adolescents may have difficulty understanding the varied personal space needs of others, and this intervention can help improve this understanding.

Instructions:

1 The professional discusses how we all need a certain amount of space between us to feel comfortable.
2 The professional models this activity with one of the group participants. The professional hands the child the end of the yarn, while the professional holds the ball of yarn.
3 The professional invites the participant to hold the yarn and walk all the way to one side of the room. The professional unrolls the yarn and walks to the other side of the room.
4 The professional and participant face each other from each side of the room. The professional explains that they will take one step forward and then stop. Other members are to watch the body language of the participant and decide if the professional is too far away, close enough, or too close. The participant then shares if the group is correct based on how they are feeling.
5 If the professional is too far away (which hopefully is the case, so take a very small step!), they will then take another step, stop, and ask members to decide too far, close enough, or too close. The participant then shares how they feel.
6 This continues until the group members or the participants say that the professional is close enough (where they will stop) or too close (where they will back up). Once the professional is at the close enough point, they will cut the string and give it to the participant.
7 Participants can work in pairs to complete this activity as described above until everyone has their own personal space yarn piece.

8 Discuss what was noticed in body language surrounding comfort and discomfort, the differences in personal space needs, etc.
9 Yarn can be brought home to help family and friends learn how much space is needed.

Processing and Application: Processing includes discussion on what group members have learned about personal space. The professional may want to ask questions related to everyone needing a different amount of personal space. This insight is important for group members to know to have appropriate physical boundaries with peers. Application of this activity can be repeated at home to ensure success.

Social Navigation Group Session Four

Length: Based on a one-hour group session.

About This Week's Group: The professional should continue to take note of any specific information they want to cover in this group session, as well as review and prep for the session. Prep would include having an alternative item (sock, for example) in case any member is uncomfortable taking off their shoe for the icebreaker. Having a general joy or sorrow ready to share and having a goodbye song ready to share. Materials for this session should be created and displayed. The ice breaker and closing activity should be practiced, and the Session Overview Form ready to give to parents.

Welcome Ice Breaker: Each group member keeps one of their shoes on and takes the other shoe off. All the off shoes go into a pile. If there are an odd number of members, the professional should put one shoe in the pile also. The therapist then mixes up the shoes and chooses a group member to go first. The first group member closes their eyes and picks a shoe. The member then finds who the shoe belongs to and asks that person a question of their choosing. The play continues until everyone has asked a question. If a group member chooses their own shoe, the professional can decide if they should try again or share one statement about themselves.

Anything to Share: The therapist should follow the same suggestions from group session one or two.

Implement the Social Navigation Intervention: The professional can use the interventions provided in this session or one of their own.

Process and Application of the Intervention: An example of processing and application is provided at the end of each social intervention description.

Goodbye Ritual: Teach the members a simple goodbye song they can sing. There are many online songs to choose from, or members can create their own.

Give Form to Caregivers: As the children leave the group session, the professional should give each caregiver the Session Overview Form. The therapist will want to have the form completed prior to the group.

Group Session Four: Example Social Navigation Intervention for Children

Activity: Symphony Composers.

Target Area(s): Including others, cooperating, working together, and executive functioning.

Level: Children.

Materials Needed: A bell set (one bell needed for each group member), color stickers, only if bells used are not a variety of colors (one color for each participant), construction paper (one color that corresponds with each color sticker or bell).

Introduction: This is a great activity to do with individuals who are not sensitive to sound. A good idea is for the professional to first be the conductor while the children get used to the idea of the game, then later they can take turns being the conductor. The focus is not on the music created but the idea of focusing, working together, and participating in a fun activity. This activity allows for structured group participation and creativity. It allows clients to have some flexibility with instrument selection but provides a safe control in a social setting. Clients can practice focus, group participation, completing a task, and other valuable social navigation methods.

Instructions:

1 The professional should have bells displayed on a table. Each group member should pick one bell.
2 Once the bells are chosen, the professional puts a different color sticker on each bell. There should be only one color of sticker on each bell that is being used. (This step is not needed if different color bells are being used.)
3 The professional lays out each corresponding piece of matching color construction paper in front of them. The professional then explains that whichever piece of paper they hold up, that corresponding bell should be played. The group may need to decide how each bell will be played (one gong, several rings, etc.).
4 The professional holds up a piece of paper and waits for the corresponding bell to play. The professional continues holding up various colors of paper until all group members have had a turn and have been successful with playing at the appropriate time.
5 Individual group members can take turns being the conductor while the professional can choose a bell to play.

Processing and Application: Processing questions can include what they enjoyed and did not enjoy about this activity. Discussion may be needed about noise volume and any sensitivities group members may have had. This could be replicated at home, either with various instruments or homemade instruments (spoons, coffee cans, dried beans put in a jar, etc.).

Group Session Four: Example Social Navigation Intervention for Adolescents

For this group day, *Symphony Composers* is a great activity for adolescents as well. The professional can modify this activity by adding a variety of instruments instead of just the bells. The professional can also allow more time for the adolescent group members to be the composers, and the group members can also video one of their songs.

Social Navigation Group Session Five

Length: Based on a one-hour group session.

About This Week's Group: The professional should continue to take note of any specific information they want to cover in this group session, as well as review and prep for the session. Prep would include having animal cards or creating them with index cards. Having a general joy or sorrow ready to share or possibly have a picture of the yoga 'prayer pose' to help with goodbye the ritual. Materials for this session should be created and displayed. The ice breaker and closing activity should be practiced, and the Session Overview Form ready to give to caregivers.

Welcome Ice Breaker: By group session, five members most likely will feel more comfortable with each other. This is a great time to introduce a fun activity like *Animal Charades*. It can be adapted for younger children by having them pick a card with an animal on it, then the group member makes noises like that animal for others to guess. With older children and adolescents, players will act out silently whatever animal card they choose.

Anything to Share: The professional should follow the same suggestions from group session one or two.

Implement the Social Navigation Intervention: The therapist can use the interventions provided for this session or one of their own.

Process and Application of the Intervention: An example of processing and application is provided at the end of each social intervention description.

Goodbye Ritual: Before they leave, group members form a circle, put their hands together (prayer pose), and give each other a bow. Group members then put their hands up to their sides, palms facing out, connect their palms with other group members, and bow.

Give Form to Caregivers: As the children leave the group session, the therapist should give each caregiver the Session Overview Form. The professional will want to have the form completed prior to the group.

Group Session Five Example Social Navigation Intervention for Children

Activity: Monster Maker.
Target Area(s): Socializing with peers, including others, and completing a task.
Level: Children.
Materials Needed: Two foam dice (the professional ahead of time writes the numbers one through six on one die; the words or pictures "eye," ""ear," "nose," "mouth," "hands," and "feet" on the other die). One piece of paper with an oval, circle, square, etc. to represent the monster's body, and one pencil for each group member.
Introduction: This is a fun activity that presents a small amount of challenge due to working with a non-realistic monster. Clients who may feel unskilled at drawing may seem more eager to attempt it when it is simple body parts to be drawn. Participants need to work on accepting the number that is rolled, taking turns on the rolling, and discussing the strengths and challenges with more or less sensory body parts than the monster has compared to them.

Instructions:

1 The professional explains that each group member will take turns rolling both dice. Once rolled, a number and body part will be shown.
2 Whatever number is rolled, the group member draws that many body parts onto the monster template.
3 Play continues until all body parts have been represented. Group members get to decide if one particular body part is rolled more than once if they roll again or keep adding that body part to the monster.
4 Group members can choose to color the monster when completed.
5 The professional leads a discussion on the strengths and challenges this monster would have with the number of each body part.

Processing and Application: Processing questions may include asking how group members felt about having to work together on this activity. Were there any new discoveries made about working in a group? What was easier to accomplish, and what was more difficult? This activity can be repeated at home with a variety of different fantasy animals and characters.

Group Session Five Example Social Navigation Intervention for Adolescents

Activity: Monster Collaborative Drawing.
Target Area(s): Socializing with peers, including others, and completing a task.
Level: Adolescents.

Materials Needed: One piece of paper for each group member, one pencil, a timer (may not be needed).

Introduction: This is a great activity for group members to learn to work with others and compromise on ideas. It also allows them to see how being flexible and part of a team can create something fun and special.

Instructions:

1 The professional will give one piece of paper and a pencil to each group member. The group members should be sitting in a circle.
2 The professional will ask each group member to fold their papers into half (top to bottom) and then into half again (top to bottom). The paper should then be opened paper should now be in four sections, from top to bottom.
3 The professional will tell each group member to draw a monster head; however, they like, in the very top section. They will want to also draw a neck that ends a bit over the second section of the paper (right past the first crease). The professional can choose to set a timer for this or not.
4 The professional will then have each group member fold the first section of the paper in the opposite direction so that the head is now hidden (but a portion of the neck can still be seen).
5 The group members will then pass their papers on to the person on their left. This time the professional will have each person draw a torso of a monster (chest, arms, hands, and stomach) on the second section of the paper. The professional will instruct the group members to have the bottom of the stomach go slightly over the crease into the third section of the paper.
6 Repeat the process of folding in the opposite direction, passing to the group member on the left and repeating, with the third section being a monster's legs, and the fourth section being a monster's feet.
7 Once the drawings are complete, open each one to see what silly monsters have been created!

Processing and Application: Discuss with the group members what they enjoyed about this activity and with what they had difficulty. Encourage them to share ways they may have struggled working in a group. Process with the group members the times and places where they will need the social tool of working in a group. This activity could be repeated at home with other types of fantasy animals and characters.

Social Navigation Group Session Six

Length: Based on a one-hour group session.

About This Week's Group: The therapist should continue to take note of any specific information they want to cover in this group session, as well as review and prep for the session. Prep would include possibly having adjective examples to help with the ice breaker activity and having a general joy or sorrow ready to share. Materials for this session should be created and displayed. The ice breaker and closing activity should be practiced, and the Session Overview Form ready to give to caregivers.

Welcome Ice Breaker: *Nifty Names* icebreaker has each group member say their name and what letter it begins with. The other group members come up with positive adjectives that begin with each group members' name. Each group member chooses the adjective they like the best and writes it on a name tag for them to wear.

Anything to Share: The professional should follow the same suggestions from group sessions one or two.

Implement the Social Navigation Intervention: The therapist can use the intervention provided for session six or one of their own.

Process and Application of the Intervention: An example of processing and application is provided at the end of each social intervention description.

Goodbye Ritual: Each group member takes a turn saying goodbye to the other group members by using each of their new, nifty names.

Give Form to Caregivers: As the children leave the group session, the professional should give each caregiver the Session Overview Form. The therapist will want to have the form completed prior to the group.

Group Session Six: Example Social Navigation Intervention for Children

Activity: Topic Tower Builders (children's version).
Target Area(s): Having a conversation, sharing with others, expressing opinions, and participating in a group.
Level: Children.
Materials: Colored blocks (around eight to ten blocks per group member).
Introduction: Neurodivergents often love to share information on preferred topics but may have difficulty including others in their conversations. This game allows each group member to share facts and opinions about animals in a more conversational, back-and-forth style. It will also encourage expressing thoughts and learning about others.

Instructions:

1 The professional puts out the tub of colored blocks and has each group member choose eight to ten. The professional tells the group that they can pick whatever colors they want.

2 All group members will sit in a circle with a sturdy surface in the middle (a surface that will allow blocks to stand on top of each other). The professional explains that they are going to call out an animal and a color. The color called out will be one of the block colors.
3 The first group member, if they have that color, will place the block down, and then say one thing related to that animal. If they do not have that color, they will skip to the next person. If they have more than one block of that color, they only put one block down and wait for their next turn.
4 Each group member continues in this matter, stacking their block onto the previous one until all the color blocks are used.
5 The game is continued, with the professional calling out an animal and a color until all blocks are used or the tower falls. If the tower falls, group members can decide if they would like to count the blocks and improve their score.

Processing and Application: Discussion can include what are facts vs. opinions, similarities, and differences between group members' statements, and how they handled waiting their turn or the tower falling. Group members can discuss where it may be important to be able to display these social navigation processes.

Group Session Six Example Social Navigation Intervention for Adolescents:

Activity: Topic Tower Builders (adolescent version).
Target Area(s): Having a conversation, sharing with others, learning about others, expressing opinions, and participating in a group.
Level: Adolescents.
Materials Needed: Colored blocks and index cards with a subject of group interest made by the professional.
Introduction: This is a great activity to allow group members to share their facts and opinions on various topics while also listening to the ideas of others. It is structured in a way that one idea is shared at a time while a block is added to the tower. Many neurodivergents enjoy sharing facts on preferred topics but may struggle discussing non-preferred ones. It can also be difficult for them to determine when to listen to their peers' comments. This activity is structured in a way that allows clients to practice discussing preferred topics one statement at a time while listening as well to what others think. It also introduces the idea of discussing non-preferred topics.

Instructions:

1 The professional creates a deck of cards, each with a topic on it. The professional needs to make sure the topics chosen are of interest to the clients and well-known to them.

2　The professional sets out blocks and subject cards. They explain that the youngest person starts first by choosing a subject card. Once a card is chosen, the player chooses a block, sets the block on the table or floor, and states one fact or opinion about the subject.

3　Play continues in a clockwise order with each player choosing a block and setting it on top of the tower while sharing one fact or opinion about the subject.

4　Each player is allowed a 'pass' if they cannot come up with a fact or opinion.

5　Each player can only share one fact or opinion at a time; no one can go twice in a row.

6　The tower is built when all passes have been used and there is no way to continue sharing without a player going twice. Blocks are counted to see how big of a conversation tower was built. If the tower falls, group members can decide if they would like to count the blocks and improve their score.

Processing and Application: Processing involves any possible difficulty with taking turns. The professional may also want to ask if there was any frustration if the tower fell. The professional may wish to review what facts and opinions are and spend some time discussing why it is important to know the difference between the two. Caregivers could practice fact versus opinion at home both in natural conversation and in game play.

Social Navigation Group Session Seven

Length: Based on a one-hour group session.

About This Week's Group: The professional should continue to take note of any specific information they want to cover in this group session, as well as review and prep for the session. Prep would include having index cards ready with each group member's name for the icebreaker and having a general joy or sorrow ready to share. Materials for this session should be created and displayed. The ice breaker and closing activity should be practiced, and the Session Overview Form should be ready to give to caregivers.

Welcome Ice Breaker: *Name Game* icebreaker involves having each group member's name on an index card. Group members pick one index card, then walk around the room finding three to five things that share the first initial with the card they chose (for example: if "Sam" is the card chosen, the child may pick up a "scarf"). Once everyone has picked items, group members have to guess which name each person had.

Anything to Share: The professional should follow the same suggestions from group session one or two.

Implement the Social Navigation Intervention: The therapist can use the interventions provided for this session or one of their own.

Process and Application of the Intervention: An example of processing and application is provided at the end of each social navigation intervention description.

Goodbye Ritual: Group members take turns hooking their pinky fingers with another group member and giving a goodbye shake.

Give Form to Caregivers: As the children leave the group session, the therapist should give each parent the Session Overview Form. The professional will want to have the form completed prior to the group.

Group Session Seven: Example Social Navigation Intervention for Children

Activity: Where It Belongs (children version).
Target Area(s): Knowing safety information, knowing appropriate hygiene, decision-making, and perspective-taking.
Level: Children.
Materials: Four pieces of construction paper hung up in each corner of the room. One piece says "home," one piece says "school," one piece says "store," and one piece says "outside" (for younger children, pictures instead of words may be more helpful).
Introduction: This activity involves movement, which can be regulating for children. The children will be thinking on their feet while moving, which can be essential in other areas of their lives. They may also encounter having to decide on one place to stand when more than one option makes sense to them. This discernment can be difficult, but practicing during game play is helpful.

Instructions:

1 The professional explains that they are going to call out something that children do. When they do, the group members should walk to the corner of the room with the sign that says the place where this would likely happen. The professional explains that there may be more than one acceptable place, but the children can choose the one that makes the most sense to them.
2 The professional then calls out up to 20 things that children do (examples include eating dessert, yelling, dancing, paying attention, taking off clothes, etc.) and gives group members time to walk to their corner.
3 The group members explain why they chose to stand where they did.

Processing and Application: Children can process with the professional why they chose to stand where they did and hear why others chose their places to stand. Discussion can include any difficulties in choosing between more than one acceptable place in the game. This game can easily be practiced at home as well.

Group Session Seven: Example Social Navigation Intervention for Adolescents

Activity: Where it Belongs (adolescent version).

Target Area: Knowing safety information, knowing appropriate hygiene, and perspective-taking.

Level: Adolescents.

Materials: Magazine pictures of places taped around the therapy room (good suggestions are bathroom, kitchen, classroom, bedroom, playground, store, doctor's office, etc.). Twenty slips of papers with verbs written on them hidden around the playroom (good suggestions are "yelling," "laughing," "whispering," "taking off clothes," "running," etc.) and tape.

Introduction: Problem-solving is an essential skill for adolescents, and adolescents may find this difficult to do in a group. Practicing working in a group is a great way to help these adolescents feel more comfortable and confident with their decision-making ability.

Instructions:

1 The professional explains that there are 20 slips of paper around the room. Group members can work individually, in partners, or in teams to find all 20 slips of paper.
2 Once all 20 are found, group members work individually, in partners, or as one team to read the verb on the slip of paper, then choose which place taped on the wall would be the best place to do this verb. If working with another person, they need to decide on one place together. They then tape the slip of paper onto the place and tell the group why they made their choice.
3 When completed, the professional makes copies of each page (with the slips of paper still on them) for each client to have their own book to take home to review.

Processing and Application: This activity allows for discussion on social navigation in a fun, game-like way. The group members may feel like they are understood and not alone in any difficulties they may have when learning from the other adolescents. The extra take-home makes for further practice on where certain activities should be done and the appropriateness or inappropriateness of certain behaviors in certain environments.

Social Navigation Group Session Eight

Length: Based on a one-hour group session.

About This Week's Group: The therapist should continue to take note of any specific information they want to cover in this group session, as well as review and prep for the session. Prep would include practicing singing the song for the icebreaker and having a general joy or sorrow ready to share. Materials for this session should be created and displayed. The ice breaker and closing activity should be practiced, and the Session Overview Form should be ready to give to caregivers.

Welcome Ice Breaker: The professional explains that every time they say a word beginning with the letter *B*, the group members are to stand if seated and sit down if standing. Then the professional sings, "Bring Back My Bonny."

> "My Bonny lies over the ocean. My Bonny lies over the sea.
> My Bonny lies over the ocean. Oh, bring back my Bonny to me.
> Bring back, bring back, bring back my Bonny to me, to me.
> Bring back, bring back, oh, bring back my Bonny to me."

Anything to Share: The therapist should follow the same suggestions from group sessions one or two.

Implement the Social Navigation Intervention: The professional can use the interventions provided for session eight or one of their own.

Process and Application of the Intervention: An example of processing and application is provided at the end of each social intervention description.

Goodbye Ritual: The professional can repeat the game *Bring Back My Bonny*.

Give Form to Caregivers: As the children leave the group session, the professional should give each caregiver the Session Overview Form. The therapist will want to have the form completed prior to the group.

Group Session Eight Example Social Navigation Intervention for Children

Activity: Move It! Move It!
Target Area: Socializing with others, regulation, and participating with peers.
Level: Children.
Materials: Foam die (the professional writes the word or picture "head," "shoulders," "arms," "hands," "legs," or "feet'" on each side of the dice) and a music source.
Introduction: Movement is an important part of regulation. This intervention is best saved for the ending group sessions since there is a degree of vulnerability with dancing. Group members by now will most likely be much more comfortable with each other. Getting in touch with their body, learning where their body is in relation to space, and moving their bodies in a variety of ways can be very helpful to clients. The idea of clients dancing in front of a group may feel intimidating, but breaking down movement in this way can feel safer and more fun.

Instructions:

1 The professional chooses music to listen to that the group members enjoy.
2 The professional rolls the die. Whichever body part is shown, that is the only body part the members move.
3 Members continue to move previous body parts, while the die continues to be rolled. If the same body part is rolled again, group members get to change up how they are moving that body part.
4 The dance is created once all body parts are moving.

Processing and Application: The professional can process with the group how they felt dancing in front of other group members. The children can be praised for their brave dancing. Movement can be discussed as an essential way to regulate when feeling worried or stressed. Invite the group members to practice some of these moves when they are feeling dysregulated in other environments.

Group Session Eight: Example Social Navigation Intervention for Adolescents

Activity: Group High Five.
Target Area: Socializing with others and participating with peers.
Level: Adolescents.
Materials: None.
Introduction: This is a whole group activity where the members form and sit in a circle. It typically works best if group members are sitting on a floor. The professional should join the circle and participate in the activity. *Group High Five* can last as long as the members want to play and can have many variations.

Instructions:

1 The professional has the group participants sit in a circle (ideally on the floor).
2 The professional explains they are going to play a game where they pass a high five around the circle.
3 The professional should begin by giving a normal high five to the person sitting to their right, and then that person continues the high five around the group circle until it gets back to the professional.
4 At this point, the professional explains that each member will send around a high five but should make a variation on the move, maybe a double high five, a pinky high five, up high, down low, with your thumbs, standing up, etc. Whatever the participant can think of, the group can do.
5 The next person to go is the person sitting to the left of the professional. This person can decide what type of high five to do and start it around the circle. Once it has gotten back to themselves, the next person can go.

6 This continues until each member has had a turn, creating a high five to send around the group circle.

7 One fun variation is to try and keep all the high fives going in unison. Another variation would be to add a reverse callout – anyone at any time can say "reverse," and the direction must change. The professional can be creative and think of many variations to this activity.

Processing and Application: Once the activity has been completed, the professional can process with the group how it felt to participate. Some processing questions might include: did you feel uncomfortable connecting with other people? What felt challenging? Was there anything about the activity that felt good or fun? Have you ever had to do anything with a group, and what was the experience like?

Social Navigation Group Session Nine

Length: Based on a one-hour group session.

About This Week's Group: The professional should continue to take note of any specific information they want to cover in this group session, as well as review and prep for the session. Prep would include possibly having picture examples of essential items for the icebreaker activity and having a general joy or sorrow ready to share. Materials for this session should be created and displayed. The ice breaker and closing activity should be practiced, and the Session Overview Form should be ready to give to caregivers.

Welcome Ice Breaker: The therapist has the children pretend that the group has been stranded on a deserted island. They must work together to come up with one item each person has that can help the group survive. This activity can be spent talking or drawing items on paper.

Anything to Share: The professional should follow the same suggestions from group session one or two.

Implement the Social Navigation Intervention: The professional can use the interventions provided for session nine or one of their own.

Process and Application of the Intervention: An example of processing and application is provided at the end of each social intervention description.

Goodbye Ritual: Since this is the second to last session, the therapist may want to take the last five minutes to discuss the group coming to an end. The professional may get ideas about celebration treats they may want or special activities they may want to do in the last session.

Give Form to Caregiver: As the children leave the group session, the professional should give each parent the Session Overview Form. The professional will want to have the form completed prior to the group.

Group Session Nine: Example Social Navigation Intervention for Children

Activity: Scavenger Hunt.
Target Area: Participating in a group, compromising, safety needs, and problem solving.
Level: Children.
Materials: None.
Introduction: This activity allows group members to problem-solve both real and imaginary situations. It can help with making choices and working with others to come to a decision. Having a visual object the participants are looking for helps make this activity easier to complete.

Instructions:

1 The professional explains to group members that any object in the room can be used for this activity (unless certain items should be off limits, for example: items on the professional's desk).
2 The professional has the group work individually, in partner groups, or as one team to choose one item in the room that would be the best used in a particular situation. Situations should be a mix of realistic and fantasy.
3 Once members have chosen the object, they explain to the professional or other group members why the object was chosen.

Examples of situations:

You need to give a gift to a three-year-old.
You need to fight a zombie.
You have a play date with a friend.
You need to fall asleep.
You must walk in the rain.
You must take a bath.

Processing and Application: Processing can occur during the activity to highlight the differences in opinion. Since the children have been processing verbally during this intervention, less time would be needed on processing after the activity.

Group Session Nine: Example Social Navigation Intervention for Adolescents

Activity: Domino Challenge.
Target Area: Working as a team, compromising, socializing with peers, and expressing ideas.
Level: Adolescents.

Materials: Colored Dominoes (the professional can use traditional dominoes that have different colored dots on each one or can purchase plastic dominoes that are a variety of colors).

Introduction: *Domino Challenge* is an excellent way to work with structure, challenge, patience, and more. Often, the dominoes fall before the track is complete, and players have to persevere and keep going. This is a great activity to also show how individual work can also be part of a greater picture.

Instructions:

1 Group members are divided into teams based on how many colors of dominos are being used (for example, if the professional has blue, green, yellow, and red dominos, there would be four teams). If the professional is using standard white dominos, they would need to add colored sticker dots to differentiate the teams.

2 The instruction is for each team to create a track of their choice with their color of dominos. The goal is to have a starting domino that, when pressed with a finger, will create a unison of the dominos falling. The team members should work together to create a domino track of their choosing (they can choose a simple straight line or can create a more elaborate path).

3 Once each team is successful with their domino tracks (meaning each team has had their dominos all fall), the new challenge is for the entire group to work together to have a large domino track with all the colors combined. Group members can decide to either stay in their teams and create connecting paths or combine all the dominos and work as one team to create the path together.

4 Once completed, the professional can tip the first domino over to see if all the dominos fall!

Processing and Application: Processing may include any frustration felt while working with the dominoes. Group members should be praised for not giving up. Examples of other times and situations where persevering may be highlighted.

Social Navigation Group Session Ten

Length: Based on a one-hour group session.

About This Week's Group: The professional should continue to take note of any specific information they want to cover in this group session, as well as review and prep for the session. Prep would include having celebration foods ready to be shared and having a goodbye take-home object for the group members. Materials for this session should be created and displayed. The ice breaker and closing activity should be practiced, and the Session Overview Form should be ready to give to caregivers.

Welcome Ice Breaker: The therapist prompts group members to think of one word to describe the ten-week group. It can be any word of their choosing (how they felt, what they learned, etc.). Each group member will share the word they chose and why they chose it.

Anything to Share: The professional should follow the same suggestions from group sessions one or two.

Implement the Social Navigation Intervention: The therapist can use the interventions provided for this session or one of their own.

Process and Application of the Intervention: An example of processing and application is provided at the end of each social intervention description.

Goodbye Ritual: The professional should have a small take-home for the group members, which can be given to them at this time. Examples include a goodie bag of candy, a photo frame with a picture of the group, etc.

Give Form to Caregivers: As the children leave the group session, the therapist should give each caregiver the Session Overview Form. The professional will want to have the form completed prior to the group.

Group Session Ten: Example Social Navigation Intervention for Children

Activity: Fill My Bucket.
Target Area: Verbally expressing feelings, connecting with peers, and empathy.
Level: Children.
Materials: The book *Have You Filled a Bucket Today?* by Carol McCloud, one small bucket for each group member (they will get to take these home), name tag stickers, permanent market, index cards, and pencils.
Introduction: This book is fantastic for every professional to have. Many schools have purchased this book for character-building lessons, so children may be familiar with it. This activity allows group members to share with each other and have a take-home object to help them remember the group.

Instructions:

1 The professional reads the book *Have You Filled a Bucket Today?* to the group members

2 The group processes the book. Sample questions include:

  a Can you give an example of how you filled someone's bucket during this group?

  b Can you think of a time where you may have taken from someone's bucket during this group?

  c Can you give an example of when someone filled your bucket during this group?

  d Is there a way we can continue to fill our group members' buckets even though the group is ending?
3 The professional gives each child a small bucket, a name tag sticker, and a permanent market. The professional asks each group member to put their name on the sticker and attach it to their bucket.
4 The professional then instructs each child to place their buckets on a table, ledge, etc.
5 The professional hands out index cards to each group member (they will need one card for each group member, including themselves.) and a pencil. The group members should write one positive thing about each group member, including themselves. It is helpful to have them first write the group member's name on the index card, so the cards don't get mixed up. The professional can help with writing if necessary.
6 The group members fill each other's buckets, placing the written index card into each group member's buckets. The professional can have the group members read during the group or at home.

Processing and Application: Termination groups can be very difficult on children, especially those who have had difficulty making and keeping friends. The professional should have extra time allotted during the group session to further process the feelings of the group terminating.

Group Session Ten: Social Navigation Intervention for Adolescents

Activity: Secret Message.
Target Area(s): Talking about feelings, sharing with others, and empathy.
Level: Adolescents.
Materials: Lemon juice, cotton swabs, white construction paper cut into fourths, markers, hair dryer.
Introduction: This activity is great for adolescents since they often get embarrassed by complimenting others or being complimented. The invisible ink gives them a level of privacy that can be important for them. This is also science-based, which many adolescents may enjoy.

Instructions:

1 The professional begins by stating this is their final group session. They allow the adolescents to process their feelings about this. Questions may include:

  a What is one positive thing you experienced about the group?
  b Is there an 'oops' you may have committed during group you would like to acknowledge and apologize for?
  c What was the most fun activity?

   d Is there something you learned being in this group?

   e Is there a way you all can stay connected even though the group is over?

2 The professional instructs the group to think about each group member and positive things about them. These can be discussed out loud or processed internally.

3 The professional gives each group member a small bowl of lemon juice, a marker, a few cotton swabs, and several pieces of white construction paper already cut into four smaller pieces. The group members will write one group member's name on each piece of paper (including themselves).

4 Group members will now write one word describing each group member using the invisible ink! They simply have to dip their cotton swab into the lemon juice, and then write the word on the paper.

5 When finished, each group member is given the papers with their names on them. Group members take turns using the hair dryer to discover each of their positive traits.

Processing and Application: Termination groups can be very difficult on adolescents, especially those who have had difficulty making and keeping friends. The professional should have extra time allotted during the group session to further process the feelings of the group terminating.

Chapter 8

Groups Examples

AutPlay® Therapy Play Groups for Children and Caregivers

Group therapy can be a valuable experience for children, providing a unique platform for relational, social, and emotional growth, peer support, and education. However, it's essential to ensure that group therapy is tailored to meet the specific needs of the children involved, with appropriate structure, supervision, and facilitation by trained professionals. Grant & Turner-Bumberry (2020) stated that the challenge for the group therapist working with neurodivergent children is to provide an atmosphere that helps children improve their happiness and success while respecting their neurodiversity. This requires mindfulness on the part of the therapist to carefully assess needs versus trying to make children "look" or become neurotypical.

Hull (2014) noted that the role of the therapist in neurodivergent-focused groups is to provide a model for group members in which they can feel safe in the relationship with the therapist as a form of learning and incorporating what they need to see in their life. Sweeney et al. (2014) furthered that the group play therapist has a crucial role in the functioning and success of the group process. There is an importance in modeling what is expected, exhibiting a belief in the process, and communicating this belief to group members.

AutPlay Therapy play groups are based on the AutPlay Follow Me Approach (FMA) in the AutPlay Therapy Framework (Grant & Turner-Bumberry, 2020). The FMA focuses on relationship development, support needs, and progression from a child's inability to focus and engage with others to participating fully in co-experienced play interventions with therapists and caregivers (Grant, 2023). The FMA is used with children who may have difficulty attuning to and being able to participate in more structured or directive play therapy interventions, as well as children too young to participate in directive processes. These children would typically not engage or interact with another person. These children may be nonverbal or limited in verbal ability and may have high support needs. While

DOI: 10.4324/9781003468370-9

the FMA approach is often used with younger children, AutPlay Therapy play groups could apply to older children or adolescents.

In FMA, the therapist and child participate in a typical play therapy room environment. The child is given no directive instructions from the professional other than a structuring statement to begin the session, such as "This is the playroom, and you can play with anything you want, and I will be in here with you." The therapist follows the child's lead, moving with the child around the playroom and trying to engage with the child in whatever activity or toy they are playing with. The professional lets the child lead but always tries to get involved in what the child is doing. The professional transitions as the child transitions and is continuously looking for opportunities to connect with the child through attunement, verbalizations, reciprocal play, or any other play and social methods.

Grant & Turner-Bumberry (2020) proposed that throughout the FMA session, the professional is using reflecting and tracking statements and being mindful of the child's comfort level. In the FMA, it is important to not only share physical space with the child but also share attention, emotion, and understanding with the child. In AutPlay Therapy play groups, the therapist is active in implementing the FMA principles as well as other group dynamics. In AutPlay Therapy play groups, the professional models, communicates, organizes, and facilitates the play group process. The therapist is both a participant and an encourager for the children and the caregivers.

In the FMA, parents work with the professional in learning how to have special play times at home with their child. Parents are taught how to have FMA play times at home with their child and thus become co-change agents in helping their child address therapy needs. Parent training and participation have been shown to be an effective and evidence-based practice when working with children. (Booth & Jernberg, 2010; Dempsey et al., 2013; Grant, 2017; and VanFleet, 2014). Neurodivergent children who have higher support needs often require more involvement from their caregivers to accomplish daily life experiences. Using the FMA framework as a guide, caregivers participate fully in AutPlay Therapy play groups. Parents participate with their child and other parents/children during in clinic group meetings as well as host a playtime meeting outside of the clinic to help further the acquisition of relational gains.

AutPlay® Therapy play groups follow an organizational format and are typically designed for high support needs of children and adolescents, those who cannot or do not engage in more structured interventions, those who may benefit from a more nondirective approach, and families that may benefit from a more nondirective playtime approach. Groups should follow the basic philosophy of nondirective and child-centered play therapy outlined by Landreth (1991), which states to establish an atmosphere of safety for the child, understand and accept the child's world, encourage the expression of the child's emotional world, produce facilitative responses, and produce reflective and tracking attention and statements. The therapist recognizes that growth is a slow process, not to be pushed, prodded, and hurried along. This is a time when the child can relax, a place where growth takes place naturally without being forced.

Group Example

A marketing invitation was advertised for participation in a ten-week AutPlay Therapy play group. After a meeting with interested participants (parent and child), an AutPlay play group was established with five parents/children. The children ranged in age from four to five years, with four of the children being male and one female. All the children had a diagnosis of autism and had been categorized as level three in the DSM criteria and significantly lacked attunement/engagement ability. Two children also had a diagnosis of intellectual developmental disorder, and one child had a communication disorder. Each parent completed the group readiness questionnaire and required forms.

Prior to the group beginning, the lead therapist met with each caregiver, and an explanation of the group process was provided regarding their participation in the play group. Scheduling was also established for parent-hosted play times for all group members, which would take place outside of the clinic setting. The in-clinic play therapy groups consisted of one lead therapist and two assistant facilitators who were supervisees of the lead therapist. All had been trained in implementing AutPlay Therapy play groups.

Prior to Session 1

All pragmatics and organizational components were established prior to group Session 1. This included meeting with each caregiver and providing them with the outline of the group meetings, having each caregiver schedule an outside-of-clinic play time and going over the expectations for the play times, compiling all members' contact information, and acquiring releases to share contact information and participate with other group members. The facilitators were mindful to make sure all members understood how the group process operated and answered any questions before the group began.

Sessions 1–4

Beginning sessions were highlighted by focusing on developing relationships and creating an atmosphere of safety and security for the children and the caregivers. Parents and children were getting to know each other better and becoming more comfortable in the group process. The play interactions were more isolated between the children and not so involved with others in the group. Most of the play in the early sessions was parallel play. This was to be expected and was a good sign that the children were becoming comfortable in this group process. It is important for the therapist to understand that the beginning session of the group may produce dysregulation for some of the children. This is a new experience with other people that can produce anxiety. The therapist is mindful of this possibility and has measures in place to help children leave the group, take a break, or access a regulating tool when needed.

The lead therapist and assistant facilitators spent a great deal of time working on engaging each of the children one on one and occasionally trying to engage children with each other. The facilitators had pre-chosen which children each facilitator would focus on in a nondirective manner – periodically providing tracking and reflective statements for those children and staying attuned to what those children were doing and expressing. The facilitators would also periodically (as it appeared naturally) attempt to play with and/or get involved in the child's play. If the child reciprocated, the play would continue. If the child was not interested, the facilitator would discontinue their attempt. This type of interaction was inconsistent in terms of happening and not happening, which is consistent with early group sessions when working with younger and higher support needs clients.

Two of the children presented as more subdued. They did not gravitate to any toys or materials and mainly sat still on one spot in the room. With these two children, the facilitators made attempts to play with them by bringing various toys and materials to them to see if they wanted to play with them. Some children may present this way due to anxiety and/or not feeling certain about what they want or can do in the group. It is important to address them with comfort and not try to force them into any situation. By the end of Session 4, these two children were more active in engaging in the playroom with various toys and materials.

The "Table" concept item was a set of foam blocks, which remained the same for sessions one through ten. For predictability, it can be helpful to choose an item for the "Table" and keep that item consistent from session to session. It is okay to change the item from session to session if the facilitators feel it is needed or would be beneficial for the group. The lead therapist and assistant facilitators worked to naturalistically engage each child in play and encourage each child to interact with other children in the group. In Sessions 3 and 4, two of the children in the group (with the assistance of one of the therapists) began to play with each other in building various items from the foam blocks on the "Table." Until Session 3, these two children had predominantly played in isolation or with their parents. By the end of Session 4, all the children but one had shown improvement in engaging with other children and some reciprocal play with the therapist and assistant facilitators.

For the first four sessions, at around the 35-minute mark, one of the facilitators went to the lobby area where the parents were waiting and instructed them to come and join the group. An important note here is that this would put 13 people in the room. Some typical playrooms may not allow for this many people to be present. It is important to think about the size of the space when deciding how many group members will participate. In the first four sessions, the parents were instructed to be present with their child and follow their child's lead in the play. The parents were also instructed to observe the facilitators as they continued to make tracking and reflecting statements and continued to try and engage in the children's play. Parents were free to ask questions, and if it was appropriate to answer in the group setting, the facilitator would respond. Otherwise, the facilitator would instruct the caregiver to remember the question, and they would address it after the group.

By the end of Session 4, several parents had improved in their ability to engage in play with their child's preferred toys and activities. The caregivers were able to let the child lead in identifying what they enjoyed manipulating and/or playing with. One parent and child were able to play various games together in the sand tray, playing together with various miniatures in the sand and putting sand into buckets and bowls. Another parent and child were able to repeatedly build towers with large cardboard bricks and knock the towers over. All parents were reporting they were experiencing play interactions with their child in ways they had not been having prior to the group involvement.

Sessions 5–6

During the middle sessions of the group therapy process, the facilitators observed a marked improvement in familiarity and comfort among the group participants (including both parents and children). The children all seemed secure in being in the group around the other members. They were all engaging in play in their own ways and having different levels of involvement with others. The parents also seemed more at ease with being in the group and navigating play with their child.

The facilitators continued to provide a nondirective play philosophy with the children and role models for the parents. The facilitators were tracking and reflecting throughout the group meeting. The facilitators were also looking for natural opportunities to engage the children in play and encouraging the caregivers to do the same. As opportunities arose, the facilitators were also attempting to engage the children with each other in various plays. All the children were navigating at their own pace and comfort level, and all the children were showing improvement in relational and connection processes.

At this point, the group had also been meeting every other week outside of the clinic for a parent-hosted playtime. The caregivers had pre-determined who would be hosting a playtime and what the location would be. Some parents chose to have this time at their own home, while others chose locations such as a park. The facilitators were checking in with the caregivers before and after each outside of the clinic play time to provide support and answer any questions the parents had. At this point, participants had experienced five to six clinic sessions and five to six parent-hosted play times. The combination of the in-clinic group sessions and out-of-clinic parent-hosted play times had greatly benefited the children and parents in forming better relationships with each other.

By the end of Session 6, the lead therapist and assistant facilitators were able to engage with and produce meaningful reciprocal play with four of the five children. They were also able to increase the engagement, acknowledgment, and play of the children with one another. Some of the parents began to work together and play with other children. During both Sessions 5 and 6 one parent had made success in interacting with another parent and child. The two children and parents were able to play a group game together using musical instruments. Another parent and child were able to share the sand tray space and join another parent and child. The children displayed the ability to engage in limited sand play together. This type of progression is not uncommon but also may not be experienced by this point in the group meetings. Children will work at their comfort level and pace. If a group facilitator is witnessing a slower pace, that is fine. It is important to move with children instead of trying to force or rush them to do something.

The parents were reporting similar results in their out-of-clinic playtimes. Several of the parents shared that their children were able to interact with each other in finger paint playtime. They would put their fingers and hands in paint and then put it on another child, touching the other child's fingers, hands, or arms. The children seemed to engage in a joint attention moment and seemed to enjoy the playtime. The parents were delighted and felt encouraged to continue to provide opportunities for interactive play during the parent-hosted play times.

Sessions 7–10

The final sessions of the group highlighted the children's growth and worked to advance the ability of each of the children in the group, giving special attention to those children who were still having challenges with engaging with others. Four of the five children were now participating regularly with the lead therapist, assistant facilitators, and/or other children in some form of interactive play. During sessions seven through ten, the lead therapist focused more attention on the one child who was not engaging as much with others to help move their progress forward. The assistant facilitators continued to engage with the other parents and children to keep advancing their newly discovered relational and play connections.

The lead therapist worked more exclusively with the more noninvolved child and their parent during the play group time to help increase the child's comfort in play and social interaction with the therapist and their caregiver. Occasionally the therapist would try to include one of the other children. During the parent and child playtime, the therapist worked with the parent to give them additional directives to help improve their child's engagement ability. By the end of Session 10, the child was showing more ease and effort to participate in some reciprocal play with the therapist and some engagement responses with one of the other children in the group. It is important to note that this child's progress is fine. There was not anything wrong with their pace. This is the movement the child was comfortable making, and efforts on the part of the therapist were done being mindful and respectful of the child's pace.

During the final session, as the group was ending their time together, it was decided that the group would continue to meet for five more sessions to give the children additional time to enhance their skills. It was also discussed that the parents would continue to meet for playtimes even after the five additional clinic groups were finished. It is fine to extend the group and allow members to exit if they wish or continue. It is also appropriate to see if group members are open to new people joining the group if there is space in the group. When a group does formally end, the therapist should discuss with the group members to continue to meet and have play times. This is a sustainable result from the group experience that is ideal.

At the end of group 10, each child in the group had advanced in their ability to play with others, engage others in a meaningful and enjoyable manner, and improve their interactions. Some children showed more growth than others, but all the children improved from the first group session and were allowed to navigate at a pace in which they were comfortable. The parents all reported positive outcomes and satisfaction with the results of the group.

Grant & Turner-Bumberry (2020) stated that the heart of AutPlay Therapy play groups has more to do with each participant's journey than any particular social/relational skill gain. The true definition of success in an AutPlay Therapy play group is the ability of a child to find comfort, hope, confidence, and success in their abilities as a social being engaging and connecting with others. The ability of neurodivergent children to experience true enjoyment in a social world that has historically represented hurt and confusion is the greatest testament to the success of AutPlay Therapy play groups. It represents the value and importance of facilitating these groups in communities across the world and providing more experiences for neurodivergent children to thrive in social relationships. The more that neurodivergent children can heal from social rejection and find a place of peace in their social world, the better off we all become. Providing safe play groups is one way that this can be accomplished. Neurodivergent children can teach us a great deal about how to appreciate and value differences and their voices must be heard. The ultimate accomplishment of AutPlay Therapy play groups is helping these children feel confident and secure in social navigation and providing the platform in which they can fully display their unique and fascinating talents.

AutPlay® Therapy Social Groups for Older Children and Adolescents

AutPlay Therapy social groups are typically incorporated with older children and adolescents who are interested in joining a group. This protocol may be implemented with younger children, but these children would need to have strengths in connection and following therapist-led group interventions. These groups, as opposed to the above-mentioned play groups, would have members participating fully in co-experienced play interventions with professionals and caregivers. Caregivers maintain an active role in these groups as well, by both attending the groups if needed and hosting play groups outside of the group setting. Although the social groups held in the professional office are directive in nature, the play groups outside the professional setting are not. These are a time when the group members can explore playing with each other in a more natural environment.

The therapist planning these social groups needs to be mindful as to the interests of the group members. Because these groups are directive in nature, the professional wants to ensure the activities planned are both fun and instructional for all the group members. If the professional does not already know the group members who will be participating, it is essential that they have at least one meeting to discover what the children enjoy doing. Although it is not mandatory, it can be very helpful to choose group members that the therapist already knows from individual therapeutic sessions.

Although the group sessions are directive in nature, there can be time allotted to the session for non-structured play and activity. In the example given below, the professional planned a 15–20-minute directive activity and then allowed for the rest of the session to be spent on free play and activity.

Group Example

In this example, the professional chose to only do group sessions with existing clients. This allowed the therapist to truly know the strengths and needs of each individual and could better place individuals together who had similar interests. Because of this, marketing was not necessary. The therapist was able to reach out to parents directly and discuss the idea of a ten-session group. The professional had three males in their caseload, two aged 11 and one aged 12. All three group members were autistic, and one was additionally an ADHD'er. All three had expressed a great desire to have friends but were having great difficulty making friends at school. One had undergone extensive bullying and was hesitant but willing to attend the group. The other two boys identified as having no friends, although one did have virtual friends, with which he played video games. He did not know their names, and they did not live by him, but he considered them friends. None of the boys went to the same school, but all three attended a public, suburban middle school. All three had their mothers as their primary caretakers; two of the mothers were single, and the children did not regularly see their fathers; the other was married, and the child had a good relationship with the father.

The professional chose these three boys to be in a group together due to several factors. For one, they were all within the same age range, and all expressed wanting a friend. They were all heavily interested in video games, especially Minecraft. They were not athletic and did not enjoy being outside. They all enjoyed building with Lego bricks and constructing with other items as well. Two of them had challenges with wanting to be in charge and at times being called "bossy." All three of them had difficulty with activities that didn't have structured rules. Their strengths included kindness and great interest in learning new things. The professional capped this group at three since the boys had limited experience navigating socially. The therapist believed that they may become overwhelmed if there were more than three in the group. The therapist also wanted to partner at times and believed the members would enjoy being able to partner with them. The parents were excited about the group and planning adventures outside of the group time. They decided they would meet at indoor places, such as restaurants since none of the boys liked being outside. The in-clinic sessions would involve the professional only due to the small number of participants as well as the professional already knowing the participants well.

Prior to Session 1

All pragmatics and organizational components were established prior to group Session 1. This included meeting with each caregiver and providing them with the outline of the group meetings, having each caregiver schedule an outside-of-clinic play time and going over the expectations for the play times, compiling all members' contact information and acquiring releases to share contact information and participate with other group members. The facilitator was mindful to make sure all members understood how the group process operated and answered any questions before the group began. The professional asked each group member to bring one special item to the first session.

Session 1

All three boys and their parents arrived on time for Session 1. The parents waited in the waiting room to get to know each other while the professional brought the three members into the playroom. All three members had previous individual sessions in the playroom, so they seemed comfortable with being in the room but were quiet since they had never been in a group before.

The group leader welcomed them to the group and invited them to sit wherever they wished. Each boy chose a beanbag to sit on. The professional then explained the group format of a 15–20-minute directive activity followed by a non-structured playtime. The therapist ensured the group members that the non-structured time could be whatever play they wanted, individual, group, or virtual play. The group leader had an iPad in the room and allowed clients to use it. If virtual play was wanted by all three, there would have to be a timer set, or the three could play together on a game. The professional explained that this session would begin with a welcome activity of learning how to say "Hello" in various languages. Provided were sheets with multiple examples.

All three were very engaged in this activity since they enjoyed learning about maps and other countries. They were then invited to say hello to the group in any language they chose, and then, if they wanted, they could share what special item they brought in and why. The professional started by showing a framed picture of a recent vacation and explained why it was special. Two of the boys stated hello in a different language but didn't want to talk about their special item. The third boy stated hello and shared about his special item. In total, this activity took about 15 minutes.

The rest of the group time was free play time, and each boy chose a different activity. Surprisingly, none chose the iPad; one chose the sandbox, one chose drawing, and the third asked to play a board game with the professional. When the time was up, we completed a short goodbye ritual of saying goodbye in Spanish (Adios). All the boys left the playroom and saw that their mothers were talking and laughing with each other. One of the boys said adios again, and the others responded in return.

Sessions 2–4

Sessions 2–4 followed the same format of a welcoming activity, a directive activity, unstructured time, and then a goodbye ritual. Session 2 continued with the hello in different languages since they enjoyed that activity. The directive activity was speaking about helpful, neutral, and harmful video game characters. Further discussion was what made these characters helpful, neutral, or harmful. The boys were very excited to discuss this and came to many agreements. Although there was a great deal of interrupting and loud voices, the professional didn't correct this. The therapist was able to see that the boys were engaged and happy, unbothered by the cadence of the conversation. It would be ableist to expect a particular way of social communication, so this was allowed since all boys were enjoying it. The activity was ended by discussing how to look for the helpful people at school and other environments. During unstructured play, the boys continued discussing the activity while also creating a war in the sand. The goodbye ritual was saying goodbye in French (Au Revoir).

Sessions 3–4

These sessions had a welcoming activity of sharing one joy and one sorrow and the same closing activity of learning goodbye in a different language. Session 3 directive activity was further discussion on neutral characters and what actually made them neutral. From this discussion, it was discovered that many times characters were neutral because there wasn't much known about them. The directive time was ended with the idea of ways to get to know neutral people at school. The professional was careful not to give any neurotypical suggestions that would not be helpful to the boys and instead listened to their ideas.

Session 4 directive activity was again focused on helpful, neutral, and harmful characters since the boys were really enjoying discussing this with a variety of anime and superhero examples. The directive activity involved how the harmful characters were dealt with in various games and whether these actions would be possible and/or appropriate in real life. This led to very animated dialogue and a lot of laughter when talking about what these dealings would look like in real life. During non-structured time during both sessions, iPad play was chosen. They each were given an allotted amount of time to be the iPad "navigator," while the other two could chime in with what to do in the game.

Sessions 5–8

By Session 5, the boys seemed to have developed a great rapport with each other. Their parents reported the play dates were going well and that they were also joining together when playing multiplayer online games. The parents stated they only needed to intervene at times when one of them would get very excited and start tapping the other two. Although this was a stim for him, the other boys did not like it and would tell him to stop. Sometimes he wouldn't, so the parent would intervene by giving examples of other ways he could stim. This did not occur in the therapy room. There were times where they would become very loud and talk over each other, but this appeared to be their way of communicating. None of them seemed upset by this, and all three of them seemed to engage in this, so there was no intervening.

All three boys liked structure and routine, so for the remaining sessions, the opening was the same joys and sorrows activity. In Session 5, they became very excited, talking about a particular joy of them all seeing a movie together. This became the directive activity for the day. It's important for professionals to remember that the goal of group sessions is discovering friendships and to feel less alone. This activity was allowing the group members to express and reminisce. Therefore, they continued talking about the movie throughout the session and acted out parts of it until the session was over. The professional invited them to say goodbye mimicking some of the characters from the movie they saw, and they enjoyed this activity, as evidenced by a great deal of laughter.

Session 6 had a directive activity in which they worked together to create a monster. The professional had one traditional die and one foam die that had various body parts on it. The therapist also had a large poster board with an oval shape on it, representing the torso of a monster. Each member took turns rolling both dice, and then drawing that many of said body parts onto the oval. Some irritation was noted when one of the members would try to roll the die while another was drawing. The professional helped navigate the situation by suggesting that the dice wouldn't be rolled until the player's drawing was finished. When all the parts were drawn, they worked together, adding stickers and coloring in the rest of the monster. The nondirective activity for Session 6 was iPad play.

Session 7 had a directive activity titled "Would You Rather?" The professional had previously created a list of questions regarding topics that interested them. Examples included: "Would you rather live in a Minecraft World or a Fortnite World?" "Would you rather have Mario or Luigi for a friend?" and more. The professional reminded the group members that it was ok for them to have different opinions and that every opinion would need to be accepted. The nondirective activity for Session7 was iPad play.

Session 8 had a directive activity called Lego World. Each member created one thing on a Lego board that they felt would be a must-have in a new community. They could then work together to create a fourth item after constructing their individual ones. The group members voted that the nondirective play for Session 8 was to continue creating a Lego world. Due to the rapport built by these sessions, the ending activity was a simple goodbye.

Sessions 9–10

The professional began working on closing activities for Sessions 9 and 10 due to the group ending after 10 sessions. The parents had expressed that they were going to continue meeting up since the boys were getting along so well, but they were still sad that the group sessions would be over. The opening activity for Sessions 9 and 10 was naming one thing that they really enjoyed about the group. The directive activity for Session 9 was created by one of the group members. He had mentioned at a previous session he thought it would be fun to have a "dance off" mimicking some of the dances from the video game they all played. They each chose one of the dances and taught it to the other group members. All of them were responsible to learn one of the dances ahead of time to teach everyone, the professionals included. This activity was so enjoyed that there was not a free play part of this session; this activity took the entire session.

The directive activity for Session 10 was reading the story "Have You Filled a Bucket Today?" The professional had bought small, plastic buckets in each member's favorite color. The therapist then had multiple-colored strips of paper in which one compliment for each group member was written on a strip and then placed in their bucket. The parents joined in on this session and wrote several kind things on strips of paper for each of the group members. They could then decorate the bucket if they wanted to with permanent markers while we had a celebration cake and drinks. We revisited saying goodbye in both Spanish and French when the session was over.

The professional reached out to all group members and parents several weeks after the group sessions to see how they felt about the group. A small questionnaire was created for the parents, and the children were orally asked the questions. All of the participants and parents believed the group was a positive experience and were looking forward to continuing play outings.

Outside-of-Clinic Play Times

The parents were able to have five play groups outside of the group sessions. Three of the play groups happened in each parent's home, which was agreed upon by all the parents. Two of the play groups happened elsewhere, one at a movie theater since a movie came out that they all wanted to see; another one was at a fast-food restaurant. The parents reported that there were no issues and that the boys all seemed to have fun together. The parents decided to continue play groups after the group was over since the boys had become friends.

AutPlay social groups can manifest in a variety of ways. The groups may have a more nondirective process or a more therapist-structured directive process. The group size can vary, and the specific play interventions utilized will depend on the preferences and interests of the group members. The essential features are that a space is created that is safe for the children to be themselves, and that relationships can develop between the therapist and the members and between the members themselves. As evidenced by the previous group example, many times friendships are formed that continue beyond the group. For neurodivergent children to enter into a space that feels unsure and leave that space having experienced a positive social relational gain is indeed a valuable gain for many neurodivergent children.

References

Booth, P. B., & Jernberg, A. M. (2010). *Theraplay.* Jossey-Bass.

Dempsey, J., Kelly-Vance, L., & Ryalls, B. O. (2013). The effect of a parent training program on children's play. *International Journal of Psychology: A Biopsychosocial Approach, 13*, 117–138.

Grant, R. J. (2017). *Autplay therapy for children and adolescents on the autism spectrum* (3rd ed.). Routledge.

Grant, R. J. (2023). *The AutPlay® therapy handbook: Integrative family play therapy with neurodivergent children.* Routledge.

Grant, R. J., & Turner-Bumberry, T. (2020). *AutPlay® therapy play and social skills groups: A 10-session model* (1st ed.). Routledge. https://doi.org/10.4324/9780367810429

Hull, K. (2014). *Group therapy techniques with children, adolescents, and adults on the autism spectrum.* Jason Aronson.

Landreth, G. L. (1991). *Play therapy: The art of the relationship.* Brunner-Routledge.

Sweeney, D. S., Baggerly, J. N., & Ray, D. C. (2014). *Group play therapy: A dynamic approach.* Routledge.

VanFleet, R. (2014). *Filial therapy: Strengthening parent-child relationships through play* (3rd ed.). Professional Resource Press.

Chapter 9

Play Interventions for Children

Activity: Find the Prize.
Target Area(s): Executive functioning, engagement, and connection.
Level: Children.
Materials: Several small prizes (candy, small toys, stickers, etc.).
Introduction: This activity helps children with various executive functioning needs as well as provides connection and engagement. The child must listen to the professional's instructions in order to find their prize. Children participate one at a time, which allows for practicing impulse control and turn-taking. The professional may have to repeat instructions and help keep children focused on the goals they are working on in this activity.

Instructions:

1 Before the group meets, the professional hides some small prizes around the group room (usually pieces of candy, stickers, or small toys, enough so there is one for each child in the group). The prizes should be hidden so they are not easy to find.

2 The professional tells the groups they are going to play a game where they try to find some prizes that are hidden around the group room.

3 The professional explains that each child will take a turn and search for a prize in the room. Once a child has found a prize, their turn is over, and the next child gets to search.

4 The child must listen to the professional as the professional gives the child directions to help them discover where the prize is hidden. The professional should give simple directions, one direction at a time that progressively leads the child to the prize. For example, a prize may be hidden in a sandtray. The professional might say, "Look for something that is rectangle shaped." "Now look for something that you can find at a beach." "Now put your hands in the thing you might find at the beach and feel around."

DOI: 10.4324/9781003468370-10

5 The professional keeps producing simple directions until the child finds the prize. At this point, that child's turn is over and another child goes next. This keeps happening until each child in the group finds a prize.
6 While a child is taking their turn, the other children are watching and encouraging.

Processing and Application: This technique presents a fun and exciting process for working on executive functioning such as focusing. It also provides a group connection as all the members are encouraging each other to find the hidden objects. Once each child has completed their turn, the professional should ask the group what the most challenging part of the activity was and what was the easiest part. The professional should also share their observations of what children seemed to struggle with and what seemed easy. The professional should ask the participants what places in their lives they must wait and it is difficult and encourage the participants to focus on being successful in those places just as they were with this activity.

Activity: The Perfect Day Collage.
Target Area(s): Self-expression and self-advocacy.
Level: Children (teens and adults may also enjoy).
Materials Needed: Paper, glue stick, markers, magazine pictures, and laptop with printer to print pictures if professional doesn't have magazines.
Introduction: Unmasking can occur when a child is able to process what their likes and dislikes are in a safe environment. This activity allows the child full freedom to create a collage based on their perfect day. The professional can give general suggestions, if necessary, but needs to be careful not to specifically state any common likes. It is important for the neurodivergent child to articulate their perfect day, not what may be a neurotypical perfect day.

Instructions:

1 The professional prepares the room ahead of time with a large piece of paper, a glue stick, and magazine photos. If photos aren't available, looking up pictures on a computer and printing them will also work. Markers should also be available in case the client would rather draw their own pictures or write instead of draw.
2 The professional begins the activity with a short explanation. An example may be Today you get to show what your perfect day would be. You can show this through pictures, drawings, or words, however you want! Your perfect day may be different from your mom's/dad's/sibling's/friend's/teacher's/etc. and that is perfectly great! This is about you and what you love. There are no rules to this; if you have one, two, or 20 things that would make a perfect day, then a perfect day it is! Let me know if you have any questions!

3 The professional provides the child with quiet so they can complete their collage. If a question is asked, the professional may answer, but no tracking or questions should be asked by the professional. It is very important for the child not to feel influenced or judged in any way.

When the client is finished, the professional may ask about the picture if the client seems interested in sharing it. This is a time when some questions may be helpful.

Processing and Application: When the client is finished, the professional may ask about the picture if the client seems interested in sharing it. This is a time when some questions may be helpful. Questions may include: tell me more about this part of your perfect day; do we think any part of this perfect day could come true; and can we share this with your parents to see if this/or part of this could happen?

Activity: Hey, That's My Personal Space.
Target Area(s): Understanding personal space and boundaries, advocacy,
Level: Children.
Materials: White paper, crayons, or markers.
Introduction: This activity helps children understand and practice personal boundaries and personal space issues. Children have the opportunity to practice with each other and the professionals. The professional should begin with a brief and simple explanation of what personal space and boundaries mean. The professional should include the participants and complete a list of personal space and boundary situations to practice. These might be situations the participants struggle with or whatever they identify. Some examples might include standing too close to others or them standing too close to you, touching others, waiting in lines, people touching you or your things, and wondering away from groups or adults.

Instructions:

1 Prior to the group meeting, the professional can create a list of personal space needs and public boundary considerations or wait and create the list with the group.
2 The professional reads and describes the list to the children.
3 The children must show the professional an example of the situations, and then show the professional how it could be handled. The children will do this through role play.
4 Each child in the group takes a turn and chooses something from the list. The professional can participate with the child in the role play, and the professional will likely have to demonstrate some solution options through the role play. Some participants may not know how to handle a situation.
5. Once everything on the list is completed, the activity is finished.

Processing and Application: Once the items on the list have all been role played, the professional should ask the participants to share if they have struggled with any of these areas. The professional can also ask the participants to talk about what they think is the hardest thing to do and what seems easy. The professional can talk about the importance of understanding boundaries and personal space when interacting with others and how to advocate for your own needs. The professional can encourage the participants to think about times and places they may be the next day when they could practice ideas that were covered in the group meeting.

Activity: Roles and Turns.
Target Area(s): Being a part of a group, playing with and supporting others.
Level: Children.
Materials: Several balls that can be tossed or kicked back and forth (preferably soft/cloth balls).
Introduction: This activity addresses multiple target areas. The participants complete the activity as a group, with each person having a role in the group. Through the activity, they practice working together as a group, taking turns, and encouraging each other. The professional may participate and role model but will certainly want to observe and make sure the participants have the opportunity to navigate on their own. This activity can be repeated several times and can be adapted to multiple variations of the same basic concept. It typically requires some space for children to move around, but one variation for limited space might be having the children sit at a table and roll a marble to each other.

Instructions:

1 The professional explains to the group they are going to be playing a game using some balls they will be throwing back and forth.
2 The professional should have a couple of balls (not enough for everyone).
3 Ideally, the children are put in groups of three. If needed, the professional can participate in a group. The professional should adjust this activity for the number of participants in the group.
4 Two of the participants in the group of three are chosen to start first by throwing the ball back and forth to each other while the third person in the group cheers for them.
5 They will do this for a couple of minutes, then the professional will say "switch" and the participants will rotate their position, so the person who was cheering now throws the ball back and forth with one of the other participants, and a new person cheers for them.
6 After about two minutes, the professional says "switch," and the participants rotate their positions again. This happens until each participant has been in the cheering position. If applicable, the activity can be repeated.

Processing and Application: The time of throwing the ball (which could also be kicking a ball back and forth or any variation) should be kept short to keep the children interested. The child in the cheering position could also be given the task of keeping track of the time. This activity can be done with other things besides balls (balloons, bubble-blowing, etc.). Once the activity has been completed, the professional should ask the group participants what it felt like to participate as a group and have specific group roles. The professional can also ask the participants to share about a time they had to do something with a group and share about what they have learned that could help them the next time they have to participate with a group of peers.

Activity: Greatness Cards.
Target Area(s): Strengths development, self-worth.
Level: Children.
Materials: Deck of Greatness Cards developed by Tammi Van Hollander.
Introduction: This intervention utilizes Greatness Cards created by Tammi Van Hollander, which consist of several cards with strengths listed on them. The cards and specific game play are implemented to help the group members identify their strengths. Tammi Van Hollander also created Greatness Sticks, which can be used instead of the cards.

Instructions:

1 The professional shows the group members the deck of Greatness Cards.
2 The professional explains that the children are going to go through the cards and make two piles. One pile is strengths they believe they have, and one is strengths they believe they do not have.
3 Once the piles are complete, the children are instructed to go through the strength pile and narrow it to ten cards they believe are their biggest strengths.
4 Once the ten are selected, the children are asked to go through the ten and select their top five. Once they have done this, the children select their top strength.
5 The professionals and group members talk about their top ten strengths and how they manifest in their lives. They also discuss their number one strength and how much that strength is activated in their life.
6 The professional and each group member then look at the pile of strengths they do not believe they have and see if there is one they would like to have as a strength in their life. If a child chooses one, the professional and child discuss how this could become a strength for the child.
7 The professional can take a picture of each child's top ten strengths and send it to the child to keep as a reminder.

Rationale: Neurodivergent children possess strengths, but often the strengths are not recognized or valued. This play intervention provides the opportunity for children to think about this concept and identify their top strengths. The strengths can be reinforced by the professional and referenced and used throughout group therapy.

Activity: Animal Pairs.
Target Area(s): Playing together, connecting, and engaging with others.
Level: Children.
Materials: Index cards and markers.
Introduction: This activity focuses on helping participants interact with others, notice others, and the beginnings of engaging with another person to get to know them better. The target areas are addressed in a fun and interactive manner using a matching game concept. The instructions use animals for the index card matching game, but anything could be chosen – toys, sports, food, video game titles, etc. If there is something that might be more engaging for the group, then the professional should choose that for the matching portion. Professionals should keep the process fun and simple, as some children may feel uncomfortable with the group's social interaction.

Instructions:

1 Prior to the group meeting, the professional will make index cards with animal names written on them or pictures of animals on them (pictures for younger children or if there are children in the group who cannot read). The professional makes two matching sets for each animal.
2 The professional explains to the group they are going to play a matching game where each participant will have to find their matching animal pair.
3 The professional passes out the index cards to the children. Make sure that everyone has a match, and make sure the children do not reveal who they are.
4 The professional will explain to the children that there is another child with the same animal, and they are going to find out who is their match by acting like the animal on their card and observing what the other children are acting like.
5 When the professional says "go," the children have to act like the animal on their card and/or make the sound of the animal on their card and find the other child who has their matching animal.
6 Once all the matches have been discovered, the activity can be played a second time with new animal index cards passed out to the participants.
7 If needed, the professional can also participate and have an animal card and try to find their match.

Processing and Application: This technique involves the whole group and has some animated and interactive elements that may be challenging for some of the group participants. The professional should be very observant of each of the participants and how they are handling the activity. Once the game has been completed, the professional should ask the group how it felt to participate in this activity – what felt comfortable and what felt uncomfortable? The professional can also ask the group to share about any times they remember interacting with others and feeling uncomfortable.

Activity: Bingo Friends.
Target Area(s): Making friends, asking questions, and getting to know others.
Level: Children.
Materials: Bingo card template and markers (Table 7.1 provides a sample bingo card).
Introduction: This activity works on engaging others, asking questions, and making friends. This activity requires the participants to interact at a fairly high level and ask each other questions. This may be uncomfortable for some participants, and the professional will want to be observant of each participant's process and assist any child who may need help. This is a fun group activity that helps children understand the processes involved in meeting and getting to know other children. The activity can be repeated in additional group meetings with the professional creating new bingo cards.

Instructions:

1 The professional will create simple bingo cards on pieces of paper before the group begins. On the bingo cards should be various identifying information about all the children in the group, such as having brown hair, being eight years old, and liking Minecraft. The card can have more squares than the number of members in the group, but each item written in a square should be something that there will be a match for with at least one of the group members.
2 The professional will share with the group that they will be playing a bingo game.
3 The professional explains that they will pass out a bingo card to each participant, and the cards will have squares on them with something written in each square.
4 When the professional says "go," the participants must interact with each other and try to find someone who matches what is written on one of the bingo card squares. One child could be a match for more than one square.
5 When they find someone who matches one or more of the statements on the bingo card, they should try to remember who it is by writing down their name on the card or some other identifying information.
6 The game continues until each participant has found a match for each square on their Bingo card.
7 Once everyone has finished, each participant can share their card, indicating who in the group they found for each matching statement on the card.
8 The professional can also participate in this activity, and there can be something written in one of the squares on the bingo card that is about the professional.

Processing and Application: This technique can involve a great deal of social interaction. If the professional is comfortable, they could participate, which might help group members feel more comfortable. The professional should ask the participants how they felt about completing this activity – what felt uncomfortable, what part was difficult, what felt comfortable, did something feel fun? The professional can also ask the participants to share about struggles they have had with meeting other children or trying to participate with other children in a group activity. The professional should also encourage the participants to think about how they could continue to practice ways to feel more comfortable meeting new people and interacting with peers in a group setting.

Meeting Places for Parent Hosted Social Groups

Arcade	Nature Center
Botanical Garden	Area Lake
Special Events (Art Fest, Cider Days, Autism Fairs)	Zoo
YMCA/Community Center	Public Pool
Discovery Center	Various Stores
Restaurants	Movie Theater
Incredible Pizza	Jump House
Sporting Event	Museum
Farms	Fair/Carnival/Circus
Amusement Park	Miniature Golf
Go Carts	Fishing/Canoeing/Hiking
Picnic	Public Library
Pottery Studio	Farmers Market
State Parks	Imax
Ice Skating Rink/Roller Skating	Road Trip
Neighborhood Walk	Mall
Church Events	Grocery Store
Pumpkin Patch	Post Office
Horse Stables	Animal Shelter

Activity: Bubbles Advocacy.
Target Area(s): Advocating for needs and understanding other people's needs.
Level: Children.
Materials: Bubbles (one bottle for every two participants).
Introduction: This technique uses bubbles to engage participants in learning how to advocate for their needs and understand other people's needs. The professional can create several different scripts or situations using a bubble-blowing process to practice advocacy. The professional should create the scripts prior to the group meeting. The scripts should address situations where the child would need to advocate for themselves.

Instructions:

1 The professional explains to the participants they are going to work on identifying and advocating for needs while blowing bubbles.
2 The professional begins by reading and demonstrating a script to use with the bubbles. The professional tells the group they are going to practice implementing the script using the bubble-blowing process.
3 The professional divides the group up into pairs and gives each pair a bottle of bubbles.
4 The professional tells the pairs to begin by blowing the bubbles and following the advocacy script. They should continue going through the script and practice until the professional tells them to stop (example scripts are provided at the end of this activity description).
5 The professional should monitor each pair and assist them if they are struggling with the script.
6 The professional should let the children practice for several minutes, and when it seems like they are accomplishing the script well, the professional can introduce a new script to practice.

Processing and Application: This activity helps children better understand advocacy efforts. The professional will likely need to conceptualize several different scripts and teach the scripts to the children, making sure the scripts are scenarios the child might encounter. Once the activity has been completed, the professional should ask the group how they felt about the activity – was there any part that was challenging, any part that seemed easy? The professional can also ask the group participants if they can think of any additional advocacy scripts the group could practice using the bubbles.

Example Social Skill Scripts

Asking a question: The participants take turns completing a whole bubble-blowing process. Someone starts as the bubble blower and will take a bottle and act like they do not know how to blow bubbles. They will ask the other person questions such as "How do I get the lid off," "How do I get the wand out?" and "How do I blow the bubbles?" The other person is in the position of answering the questions. Once the blower completes all the steps and blows some bubbles, they switch roles.

Telling others you don't like something and hearing them tell you they don't like something: One person blows the bubbles; the other person says, "I don't like bubbles, please don't blow them by me." The bubble blower says, "Sorry, I will blow them over here." Then the other person says, "okay." They switch roles and practice this script back and forth several times.

Activity: An Emotional Story.

Target Area(s): Executive functioning, identifying emotions, and perspective-taking.

Level: Children.

Materials: None.

Introduction: This activity helps children work on executive functioning needs by focusing on keywords or phrases related to emotions. It also helps children identify when someone is experiencing an emotion and why another person might be experiencing a certain emotion. The professional creates one or more short stories that the professional will read to the group. The stories should have multiple examples of emotions being felt.

Instructions:

1 Before the group meeting, the professional will write one to three short stories that reference people feeling various emotions (some examples are provided at the end of this activity description).

2 The professional explains to the group that they will be reading a short story, and they are going to try and focus their attention on specific things in the story.

3 The professional explains that while they are reading the story, the group needs to listen, stop the professional, and identify every time an emotion is expressed in the story.

4 The participants must state what emotion is expressed, who in the story is expressing the emotion, why the person in the story is expressing the emotion, and if they would feel that way in the same situation.

5 These are questions that can be asked by the practitioner each time a child stops the story to identify an emotion.

6 After the story is finished, the professional can read another story or ask the participants if they want to write their own emotional story. If the participants write their own emotional story, they can then read the story and have the other group members identify the emotions.

7 When reading the story to the group, it is likely the participants will miss some emotions. The professional should stop the story and mention to the participants that there was an emotion they missed and re-read that section of the story to provide the group an opportunity to identify the missed emotion.

Processing and Application: This activity works on identifying emotional experiences as well as perspective-taking regarding emotions. The difficulty and length of the story should vary depending on the group members' ages and awareness of emotions. Several different stories can be written, referencing many different situations. Children who struggle recognizing the emotions in the story may need to start by reading the story themselves, circling all the emotions they find in the story, then discussing the emotions. Once the activity has been completed, the professional should ask the group to share how they felt about the activity – was it easy to notice the emotion, or was it challenging to stay focused and listen? The professional can also ask the group members to share what they think is the most challenging thing they do, where they must stay focused and listen.

Example Emotional Story 1 – Sam's First Day of School

Sam was awakened by his alarm clock. It was 7:00 am and time to get up and get ready for the first day of school. Sam was feeling tired and really didn't want to get out of bed. Sam's mother told him he had to get out of bed and get dressed; she was worried he would miss the school bus. Sam got out of bed and started getting dressed. Sam was excited to see some friends he had not seen all summer but anxious that there might be a bully at school. Sam got dressed and ate his breakfast, which gave him a sick feeling in his stomach. Sam continued to feel anxious as he got on the school bus. There was a lot of noise on the bus, and Sam was getting irritated by all the loudness. The bus finally got to school, and Sam went into his classroom. Sam was feeling relieved to finally be at school. Sally, one of Sam's best friends, came and sat beside him; this made Sam happy, and he thought maybe school was not so bad. Sam actually started to feel excited about going to school this year, even if it meant he had to get up at 7:00 am every morning.

Example Emotional Story 2 – Sally's Brother

Sally walked into her room ready to play with all her toys and have a lot of fun! As she walked into her room, her mood changed from excited to angry! Sally's little brother Michael was in her room, and he had broken several of her toys. Sally was so angry that she yelled at the top of her lungs for Michael to get out of her room. Michael seemed surprised and scared at the same time. Michael quickly ran out of Sally's room. As Sally looked around her room, she felt sad, many of her favorite toys were broken. Sally's mother heard Sally yell at Michael and came into Sally's room. She saw Sally looking sad and upset and realized what had happened. Sally's mother told Sally that everything would be OK; they would replace all the toys that had gotten broken. Sally started to feel happy. Sally's mother also told Sally that they would get a special lock for her door so her brother could not get in. Sally was excited to get some new toys and relieved that her brother would not be able to get in her room.

Activity: Together Balloons.
Target Area(s): Teamwork, communication and strategy, and connecting with others.
Level: Children.

Materials: Balloons (one for every two group members).

Introduction: *Together Balloons* provides a simple, fun, and engaging way for group members to work on connecting with each other, working together to accomplish a task, and having fun together. The professional will want to make sure that no group members have an allergy to balloons or have a fear of balloons. This should be discovered prior to the group meeting, and if there is a member with one of these issues, then this activity should not be implemented.

Instructions:

1 The professional explains to the group members they will be playing a game together that involves a balloon.
2 The professional explains they will be dividing up into pairs, and each pair will have a balloon. The professional can choose the pairs and should place the children with their partner at this time.
3 The professional blows up the balloons (or may already have them prepared) and explains to the children they are going to work together with their partner to keep the balloon in the air and not hitting the ground. They are working as a team, and they should help each other.
4 The children stand facing each other and grab each other's hands and hold both hands in front of them. The professional explains that they must keep holding each other's hands the whole time while they are trying to keep the balloon in the air.
5 If the balloon hits the ground, it should be picked up and the game started again. The activity should be played for several minutes, then the children can switch pairs and play again.
6 The professional should make sure the children understand the activity is about having fun and not mastering keeping the balloon in the air. It is likely the balloons will hit the ground often.

Processing and Application: This technique helps children work on connection and relationship development through physical touch, working cooperatively, and attuning to and being aware of others. The professional should decide how long to play the activity and how often to switch pairs. Once the activity has ended, the professional should process with the members and ask them how they felt about the activity – was there any part of interacting with another person that was challenging, was anything easy? The professional can also ask the group participants to share about a time when they had to work with another person and what that experience was like.

Activity: Boatman.
Target Area(s): Executive functioning, working together, and playing with others.
Level: Children.

Materials: None.

Introduction: This technique helps children practice playing an organized game with a group of peers. The children also work on focusing and cooperation skills. The professional may participate in this game and will want to clearly go over the game rules to make sure everyone understands what they are doing. This can be a very fun and exciting game with a great deal of social interaction; thus, the professional will want to carefully monitor the participants to make sure they are managing the activity well.

Instructions:

1 The professional explains they are going to play a popular children's game called Boatman.
2 One child is chosen to be the boatman (catcher). The boatman stands in the middle of the room. The rest of the group participants choose to stand on one side or the other of the boatmen. If no one wants to be the boatman, the professional can start by being the boatman.
3 When the professional says "go," the group members say together, "Boatman, boatman may we cross the river?" The boatman then answers, "Only if you are…" and then describes a category such as "…wearing blue."
4 The boatman's choice of category can be as general or specific as they wish.
5 All the members who meet that category must run and cross the river to the other side without being caught. The boatman tries to touch them as they are trying to get past the boatman.
6 Any children who are caught join the boatmen in the middle and help with the catching.
7 The process repeats until all the members have been caught, then a new group member can be the boatman and the game can be played again.

Processing and Application: If there is time in the group meeting, each group participant can take a turn as the boatman. If a child does not want to be the boatman, they should not be forced into that position. Once the activity has been completed, the professional should ask the members to share how they felt about playing with others in an organized game. The professional can also ask if they have ever had this type of experience before and what it was like – did it go well, was it challenging?

Activity: Safe and Unsafe.
Target Area(s): Safety skills, being mindful, executive functioning.
Level: Children.
Materials: Paper or cardboard for each group member, and markers or pens.
Introduction: This activity focuses on helping children learn about safe and unsafe situations and behaviors. The professional is encouraged to make the

activity as fun and engaging as possible. It is most helpful if the professional knows about some behaviors that group members have been doing that are unsafe and targets these behaviors in the scenarios.

Instructions:

1 The professional explains to the group they are going to do an activity that focuses on learning about safe and unsafe things and behaviors.
2 The professional gives each child two pieces of paper or two pieces of cardboard. The pieces should be square pieces, approximately 4 × 4.
3 The participants are instructed to write an S on one piece and a U on the other piece, and the children can decorate the two pieces however they want. The S stands for safe and the U stands for unsafe.
4 Once the participants are through decorating their S and U cards, the professional tells them that they are going to give them scenarios or situations and they have to hold up their S card if they think it is safe or their U card if they think it is unsafe.
5 The professional provides several scenarios and tries to match the scenarios to issues the group members might be experiencing.
6 Once the professional has finished, they can ask the group members if any of them want to share situations or scenarios and have the rest of the group respond with their safe or unsafe cards.

Processing and Application: At any point in this activity, the professional may need to stop and elaborate more on why a situation or behavior would be unsafe. Some children may have questions or may not understand why a situation would be unsafe. These questions should be addressed by the professional. Once the activity has been completed, the professional should ask the members if they have any questions about the activity or any questions about safe and unsafe behaviors.

Example Situations and Behaviors

- Crossing a street without looking for cars.
- Playing a video game.
- Running across a parking lot.
- Getting into a car with a stranger.
- Eating at a restaurant.
- Wading out into a pond or lake.
- Reading your favorite book.
- Running away from your parents in a store.
- Feeding your pet fish.
- Talking to someone you don't know online.

- Talking to your grandma on the phone.
- Running away from home.
- Petting a strange dog or other animal.

Activity: Progressive Balloon Game.
Target Area(s): Working together as a team, engagement and connection, and regulation.
Level: Children.
Materials: Balloons (one for every two participants).
Introduction: This activity can be done in pairs or in groups of four. It is a cooperative game where the participants must work together to keep a balloon in the air. The participants must progress through four levels, with each level increasing in difficulty. Before implementing this activity, the professional should make sure none of the participants have a balloon allergy or a fear of balloons.

Instructions:

1 The professional explains they will be playing a game using balloons.
2 The professional divides the group into pairs and gives each pair a blown-up balloon.
3 The game has four levels and much like a video game, the pair must progress through each level and each level gets progressively more difficulty. The pair must work together as a team to keep the balloon from hitting the floor.
4 The professional begins by telling the participants to hit the balloon back and forth any way they like and keep it from hitting the floor (this level is not difficult, and most children will be able to do this very easily).
5 After a few minutes, the professional tells the participants to grab their balloons, and now they will be progressing to the second level. At this level, the participants must take their dominant hand/arm and put it behind their back – they cannot use it. The participants begin hitting the balloon again with the objective of keeping it from touching the ground.
6 After a few minutes, the professional tells the participants to grab their balloons, and they have all progressed to the third level. In this level, both hands/arms are put behind the back and cannot be used. The participants can use their feet, knees, and heads. This level will be more challenging, and some of the participants may have their balloons hit the ground. The professional should tell the children to pick their balloons up and keep going if they hit the ground.
7 After a few minutes, the professional tells the participants to grab their balloons, and they have all progressed to the final fourth level. At this level, the participants can only use their heads. They should try to hit the balloon back and forth ten times without it touching the ground. After the participants

have played this round for a few minutes, the professional can stop the activity.

8 The professional can combine pairs and have one large group going through the progression using two or three balloons. This activity should be fun and not competitive. The professional will want to encourage the children to have fun, work together, and support each other.

Processing and Application: Once the game has finished, the professional should ask the group how they felt about working with another person to keep the balloon in the air – was there anything that was difficult, was there anything that seemed easy? The professional should ask the participants if they can think of other situations where they had to work with someone else to accomplish something.

Activity: Midline Mirror Moves.
Target Area(s): Connecting and engaging with others, executive functioning, and regulation.
Level: Children.
Materials: None.
Introduction: Midline crossing moves have been demonstrated to cross the midline in the brain and help children improve focus and concentration, reduce anxiety, and increase regulation. This activity combines a common connection intervention, the mirroring game, with midline crossing moves. The benefits of this activity include helping children increase engagement and connection with others while working on improving regulation ability.

Instructions:

1 The professional will have the group members stand up so that each member has some open space around them. The professional will stand in front of the group so each member can see the professional.
2 The professional will tell the group they must follow the professional's movements and mirror what the professional is doing.
3 The professional will then begin doing different movements, and the participants will mirror. The professional should not move too fast, and they will want to regularly create midline crossing moves. A midline crossing move is any movement where the body crosses, such as a body hug or tapping the elbow to an alternate knee. Every move does not have to be a midline move, but several of the movements should cross the midline.
4 The professional can decide how long they want to continue the mirror midline activity.
5 Once the professional is finished, they can ask if there is anyone in the group who wants to lead the group in some more midline mirror moves. Any member who would like a turn should have the opportunity.

6   Another variation would be to have the group members pair up and each pair take turns doing the mirror midline moves to each other.

Processing and Application: This group activity can last as long as the professional and the members want to keep playing. Once the activity is over, the professional should process with the members if there was anything that felt uncomfortable or challenging about the activity. The professional may want to ask members how it felt to follow another person and, depending on the variations performed, what it felt like to do the activity as a whole group versus one on one with a partner.

Activity: Animal Feelings.
Target Area(s): Emotion recognition, body awareness, and regulation ability.
Level: Children.
Materials: None.
Introduction: *Animal Feelings* is a fun and interactive activity that can be silly while helping children recognize different feelings and how those feelings may manifest. Some neurodivergent children may have a difficult time identifying and understanding their emotions and how to express the emotions they are experiencing. This activity can be played repeatedly if the members want to keep playing.

Instructions:

1   The professional instructs the children to stand around the room.
2   The professional explains they are going to play a game called *Animal Feelings*.
3   The professional tells the children they will be naming an animal and putting a feeling with the animal. The children must act like that animal and express their feeling as they think that animal would. For example, the professional might say "Angry bear," and all the children then act like a bear who is feeling angry.
4   The professional allows the children to act like the feelings animal for around one minute and then calls out a new animal feeling. The professional should go through several animal feelings.
5   Some examples of animal feelings include shy rabbit, excited fox, sad elephant, happy goat, worried chicken, proud lion, etc. The professional can make up several animal feelings and even change them up in the activity – there can be multiple happy or sad animals.
6   Once the professional has named a few animals, they can ask the group if any of the children want to lead in calling out animal feelings. Each child can have a turn if they want.

Processing and Application: Once the technique has been completed, the professional should have the group sit in a circle and ask them how it felt to complete the activity. The professional will want to ask how it feels to try and identify different feelings and if that is something the children do well in their daily lives. Some processing questions might include: did you feel comfortable trying to express all the feelings? Were some harder than others? Did you notice anything about other children's feelings? And how do you think you could express your feelings in your daily life?

Activity: Volcano.
Target Area(s): Emotion identification and regulation.
Level: Children.
Materials: None.
Introduction: Neurodivergent children may struggle with regulation and easily become dysregulated, which can often lead to an out-of-control system. This technique introduces children to understanding how dysregulation, frustration, and feelings of being upset can grow in a person and lead to a behavior explosion. It presents the concept in a fun and experiential method that can be replayed multiple times.

Instructions:

1 The professional has the children stand around the room and explains to them that they will be playing an activity called *Volcano.*
2 The professional explains they will be taking the children through a guide of expressing how a volcano grows and explodes. They will be using their bodies to express the growing and exploding volcano.
3 The professional has the children get into a crouching position and grab their knees with their opposite hands. The professional tells the children they are volcanoes.
4 The professional then takes the child through a progression – the professional says
    "You are a volcano that is starting to get restless, start moving your body just a little bit." "You are now getting more uncomfortable, move your body more and start to move your body out of the crouching position."
    "Your volcano is now building more, you are getting more upset, move your body where you are now standing and your hands are to your side – continue to move your body around, shake a little bit."
    "You are now getting very upset and getting ready to explode. Jump up and down a bit and move your body around more aggressively."
    "You have now reached explosion! Jump around, move around the room, move quickly and wildly!" "You are exploding everywhere and there is no control!" The professional should become more animated with this instruction. The children should stay in their explosion state for 20 seconds and the professional should make sure everyone is safe as they are "exploding" around the room.

5 After around 20 seconds in the volcano explosion state, the professional should instruct the children to slow down and come back to a crouching position and repeat the whole process. The process should be completed a few times.

Processing and Application: After completing the volcano activity a few times, the professional should have all the children sit in a group and do some processing questions. The professional should begin by explaining that the volcano example illustrated how we can get dysregulated in our bodies and how the dysregulation builds to a behavior explosion. Some processing questions include: have you noticed how upset feelings have built in you and then you "exploded?" What does it look like in your daily life when there is an explosion? And what are some ideas to help you stop the building and not reach an explosion?

Activity: Sword Balloons.
Target Area(s): Interacting (playing) with another person, competing (winning and losing), self-awareness, and regulation.
Level: Children.
Materials: Pool noodles (two) and balloons (one for every two participants).
Introduction: This technique uses pool noodles (as swords) and balloons to engage children in a fun and interactive activity, which helps them learn to be more comfortable playing with another person in an organized game. It also works on helping children accept winning, losing, and general rule play. The sword and balloon action helps increase self-awareness and regulation. Pool noodles are suggested for swords as they are soft and likely not to hurt if someone is accidentally hit.

Instructions:

1 The professional has the children get into pairs and gives each child a pool noodle sword and one balloon (blown up and tied off) for the pair. Each pair will need a bit of space from other pairs to ensure that children do not accidentally hit other children with their swords.
2 The professional tells the children they are going to battle each other in a game of sword balloons.
3 The professional will say when to start, and then the pair hit their balloon with their pool noodle swords. They are trying to hit the other person with the balloon. They cannot hit each other with their swords. The swords are used to hit the balloon toward their partner and to try and hit their partner with the balloon. They also cannot hit the balloon with their hands; they can only hit the balloon with their swords.
4 Often, children will accidentally hit themselves with the balloon, and this counts as a hit. The game can get very lively and should stay focused on having fun.

5 Once someone has been hit five times with the balloon, the game is over, and they can play another round.
6 The professional should monitor each pair to make sure children are not becoming frustrated, manage any disagreements, and keep the game focused on having fun.

Processing and Application: The technique should be played for around 15 minutes, and then the professional will have the children come together as a group for some process time. The professional should ask the group participants how it felt to play this game and interact with another person. What felt fun, easy, and challenging about it? The professional should ask the group members to share about times in their daily lives when they had to interact with or play with another person, and how did it go?

Activity: WRJMD.
Target Area(s): Working (playing) as a group and regulation.
Level: Children.
Materials: None.
Introduction: WRJMD stands for walk, run, jump, march, and dance. This activity is a fun group activity that provides the opportunity for children to participate together as a group and help develop regulation ability. The acronym and the specific moves can be changed. Other options might include skipping, hopping, crawling, stomping, etc.

Instructions:

1 The professional has the group participants stand somewhere in the room.
2 The professional explains they are going to play some fun music and then give the participants a specific move to do to the music. This activity does not require music. If the professional does not have access to music or if there are participants who have a music sensitivity, music does not need to be played.
3 The professional will change the move after about one to two minutes.
4 Using the WRJMD acronym, the professional will start by asking the participants to walk around the room. After about one to two minutes, the professional will switch to run around the room; after one to two minutes, switch to jump around the room, then march, and lastly dance around the room.
5 Once the activity has been completed, the professional can take the participants through the activity again, playing a different song.

Processing and Application: This technique should not last longer than 20 minutes. Once it has been completed, the professional should have the group members come together for processing. The professional should ask the members how it felt to participate in this activity with each other. Some additional processing questions might include: have you ever participated in a fun group activity in your daily life and how did it go? Also, the professional can ask the participants what felt good and not so good completing the activity and process through their responses.

Activity: Group Machine.
Target Area(s): Completing a task with a group, teamwork, engagement, and communication.
Level: Children.
Materials: None.
Introduction: *Group Machine* gives participants the opportunity to work together as a group and accomplish a task. The process is designed to be fun and engaging and allow the children to feel empowered in working together, communicating, and achieving a task. Some neurodivergent children struggle in group formats, especially when working with a group to complete a task. *Group Machine* is an engaging activity to help neurodivergent children feel more confident and successful when navigating groups.

Instructions:

1 The professional shares with the participants that the group is going to be working together to complete a task. If you are seeing a large group (eight to ten participants), you may want to create two groups instead of one large group for this activity.
2 The professional explains that the group is going to create a machine using their bodies. Each person in the group will be a part of the machine that is created. The professional should present the activity in a fun and playful way, encouraging the group to have fun with the activity.
3 The group must decide what machine they are creating and what part of the machine each person will be.
4 The machine should have a name and a purpose.
5 The group must also design how each part of the machine (each person) connects physically together.
6 Once the group has finished their design, they will present the machine to the professional. One person will introduce the machine (name and what it is for), and then each person will connect to each other one at a time and say what part of the machine they are.
7 This is a higher-level activity for group members. It may challenge some of the members with social interaction. The professional should monitor the process and assist the group if needed. The professional should observe for communication, decision-making, working together, each person contributing, and making sure the members are not becoming too anxious or dysregulated by the activity.

Processing and Application: Once the group has finished presenting their design, the professional asks the group to sit in a circle for some processing time.

The professional should ask the participants what it felt like to work together as a group to create the machine. Additional processing questions could include: what part was hard for you? What part was easy? And have you ever worked with a group before to accomplish a task? The professional should share any observations they had watching the group process and ask any questions they might have about what they observed.

Activity: Backward Moves.
Target Area(s): Participating in an activity with a group, and regulation.
Level: Children.
Materials: None.
Introduction: This activity provides a fun and interactive game that the whole group plays together. The professional facilitates a series of moves that the group members must complete backward. The moves the professional presents include walking, hopping, moving in slow motion, swimming, dancing, crawling, etc., all done backward. Participants must navigate around each other and follow instructions presented by the professional. This activity also helps improve regulation ability.

Instructions:

1   The professional has the group members stand around the room.
2   The professional explains they are going to complete a group activity where the professional will call out different moves to do and the participants must do the moves backward.
3   The professional should be sure to explain that participants should be aware of each other and try to avoid running into each other.
4   The professional begins by telling the participants to walk around the room backward. After one to two minutes, the professional says to hop backward around the room. After about one to two minutes, the professional says to walk quickly backward, then act like you are swimming backward, then move in slow motion, then dance, and lastly crawl backward. The professional can add additional moves if they would like.
5   It's also fun to add having the group try to pronounce different words backward, such as think of how to say the word play backward, then give a countdown, and have all the group members try to pronounce the word backward in unison.

Processing and Application: Once the activity has been played, the professional can have some processing time with the group. The professional can begin by asking the members how it felt to play the activity together and if there was anything that was challenging. The professional can also ask the members what their experience has been playing with peers in a group activity or game. The professional will also want to share any observations they had watching the group interaction.

Chapter 10

Play Interventions for Adolescents

Activity: Bubble Tag.
Target Area(s): Cooperation, working together as a group, and communication.
Level: Adolescents.
Materials: Bubbles (one bottle for every member of the group).
Introduction: This activity involves the whole group playing together. Bubbles are used to play a game of tag, and throughout the course of the game, each child is working on a team trying to achieve a common goal. It is most helpful to play this game in a small- to medium-sized space with some boundaries. This activity is also very fun and lively. Once the game has been played, it can be repeated several times.

Instructions:

1   The professional tells the group they are going to play a game of tag using bubbles.
2   The professional explains that there will be two participants who will be given bubbles, and they are the taggers. They must tag other group members by blowing bubbles and touching the other participants with bubbles (they do not tag or touch them with their hands).
3   The professional establishes what the boundaries are of the room (where participants can move around).
4   The professional gives each tagger a bottle of bubbles and tells the group they can begin. If someone gets touched by any bubble, they then get a bottle of bubbles and join the taggers trying to get the rest of the group.
5   This continues until everyone in the group has been tagged.
6   The professional can participate and start out being a tagger.
7   This activity usually does not take long to complete. It can be repeated several times.

Processing and Application: This is a whole group activity, and regardless of what is happening, each child is always part of a group with a common purpose.

DOI: 10.4324/9781003468370-11

It provides a fun and engaging way for the group to play together and experience being together in a social game. Once the activity has been completed, the professional should ask the group members how it felt to participate in the game. The professional should ask the participants to share about any part of the activity that felt uncomfortable or challenging.

Activity: Me and My Strengths.
Target Area(s): Strengths development, self-worth.
Level: Adolescent.
Materials: Paper, markers.
Introduction: Neurodivergent adolescents may have never been introduced to the concept of strengths and do not understand that they have strengths. This is an expressive (drawing and coloring) intervention that helps adolescents identify strengths.

Instructions:

1 The professional gives each group member a piece of paper and markers or crayons.
2 The professional explains that they are going to work on identifying strengths.
3 The professional asks each member to draw an outline of a person on their paper, covering most of the paper.
4 The professional asks each member to draw their own face and hair on the person.
5 For the rest of the person, the adolescents are instructed to think about different strengths they have (the professional can help identify strengths), give each strength a color, and color it in their person somewhere.
6 Group members can have as many strengths as they can think of, and they can indicate any type of strength.
7 Once the person is completed, the professional asks the members to share their strengths; what strength goes with each color and why they believe they have this strength.
8 The professional will want to encourage the adolescents about their strengths and have them take their strengths person home to keep and reference.

Processing and Application: Helping neurodivergent children recognize and appreciate their strengths can be an ongoing progress. This play intervention provides an opportunity for group members to identify and talk about their strengths and keep the person they created as a reminder of their strengths. Remembering and appreciating strengths will likely be an ongoing theme, and other strengths-focused interventions can be revisited and completed in different group meetings.

Activity: Teach Me-Virtual Version.
Target Area: Self-Esteem and Self-Advocacy.
Level: Adolescents.
Materials Needed: Gaming device, paper, and pen for the professional.
Introduction: Neurodivergent adolescents may feel as if they are constantly being taught to be a certain way, and this can be exhausting. Many adolescents are skilled at video games, and neurodivergent adolescents are no exception. Adults are often critical of gaming and may unintentionally shame adolescents about their use of playing. This can be harmful for adolescents since they often feel a sense of achievement and positive self-worth from gaming. In this activity, the professional asks in a previous session if the adolescent would be willing to teach the basics of a particular video game. If the adolescent agrees, the next session will be spent with the adolescent teaching the professional.

Instructions:

As discussed in the introduction, the professional has already asked the adolescent if they are willing to teach the professional a particular game. This activity is only completed if the adolescent seems excited to do this.

1 The professional has the gaming system set up to the agreed-upon game, or the client brings in their gaming device. The professional gives any directives they feel necessary to help them learn. Examples include:

   a "Gaming is a challenge for me, are you ok if I ask a lot of questions?"
   b "Can I ask questions at any time, or will you set aside a time for questions?"
   c "Are you o.k. if I write down what you are doing so I can understand better?"
2 The adolescent then plays the game with the professional next to them. They both need to be able to view the game. The profession then follows whatever was agreed upon prior to playing.

Processing and Application: Processing may occur throughout game play. Many clients will become very excited about teaching me something they love, and they can be very expressive. The professional should keep a clipboard with notes and write out questions for the adolescent after they have finished playing the game. The professional and client can also have agreed-upon stopping points throughout the game play, for the professional can ask questions, or they can explain what they were doing in the game. Some adolescents may want to teach the professional how to play throughout the process. Some professionals may not be well versed in video games, and many adolescents can show great empathy in teaching the professionals. This is something the professional can bring up when the gaming session is over. The professional can point out specifics of what they needed to learn and how openly the client taught them. The professional should try to process with them how they deserve the same empathy when trying to learn.

Activity: Keep It Going.
Target Area(s): Cooperation, completing a group task, and relationship development.
Level: Adolescents.
Materials: White piece of paper (one for every two participants) and pencils.
Introduction: This activity is completed in pairs and focuses on playing and completing a task together. As the name implies, the activity can be played until the participants are no longer interested. It does require drawing, but it is not necessary to be a "good" drawer to participate in the activity. Professionals will want to stress this point to the group members before beginning the activity.

Instructions:

1 The professional explains that the group will be completing an activity by working in pairs.
2 The professional should divide the group members into pairs, and the professional can participate if needed.
3 The professional gives each pair a white piece of paper, and each person gets a pencil.
4 The professional states that one person will start and draw a simple squiggle or line somewhere on the piece of paper. The other person then must take the squiggle or line and turn it into a picture of something.
5 The pictures are typically simple and sometimes silly. The drawing does not have to be elaborate or even accurate.
6 Once the person is finished turning the squiggle into a picture of something, the person draws a squiggle or line somewhere on the paper, and then the other person has to turn that squiggle or line into a picture of something. This keeps going back and forth until the participants are no longer interested in playing.
7 Typically, a white piece of paper will be full of eight to ten drawings by the time the activity ends.

Processing and Application: When it seems like the participants are no longer interested in keeping the drawing activity going, the professional can end the activity. The professional will want to process with the group what it felt like to work and play with another person in this capacity – what was challenging and what felt okay? If there is time, the professional could have the group members rotate playing this activity with each member of the group to create different social experiences.

Activity: Circle Picture.

Target Area(s): Cooperation, working in a group, and executive functioning.

Level: Adolescents.

Materials: Large piece of paper, pencils, colored pencils, compass, or circle templates (circle templates can be found at art supply stores).

Introduction: This activity allows group members to create art together but challenges them by having to take turns and creating only one piece of artwork. Circles can be relaxing shapes to draw, which may help individuals while working within the group.

Instructions:

1 The professional gives each group member a pencil. The group members sit in a circle with a large piece of paper in the center.
2 The professional starts by taking a compass or a circle template and drawing one circle anywhere on the paper. The professional then explains that each group member will get to do the same. They also explain that circles can overlap each other and be placed anywhere on the paper.
3 The paper is passed clockwise, with each group member choosing a circle size and drawing a circle on the paper. Paper can continue to be passed around to where each group member gets two or three turns drawing a circle.
4 When the drawing is complete, the professional can have the group members color in the circles, or parts of the circles since there may be overlapping. The professional should be more directive with this part of the activity if they feel the group members cannot complete this activity successfully (for example, assigning each group member part of the page to color).

Processing and Application: The professional may ask the group questions at the end of this activity, including: how did it feel creating circles the first time/second time/third time? Was it easier or more difficult the second/third time? Explain why? What did you enjoy about this shared artwork? What was a challenge? Did the artwork turn out how you thought it would? How is working in a group different than working alone? What did you need to practice to make this activity successful? Are there other times/places/activities where you have to work in a group? How can you use what you practiced here in those situations?

Activity: Color by Number Picture.

Target Area(s): Cooperating, working together, perspective-taking, and executive functioning.

Level: Adolescents.

Materials: Have a simple mandala printed. The professional should lightly place a number into each part of the mandala; the number should correspond to the total number of group members. This activity also needs a bucket of crayons.

Introduction: This is an artistic activity that is also low pressure for group members. The mandala is already drawn, so it simply needs to be colored in. This activity not only allows group members to color using their favorite color but also challenges them to accept the favorite colors of other group members. There is an additional challenge to take turns and follow the directions.

Instructions:

1 The professional has each group member pick their favorite color from a bucket of crayons.
2 The professional then assigns each group member a number from 1 to ___ (the largest number is a total number of group members).
3 The professional has the group members sit in a circle and places the mandala in the center of the circle. The professional shows them how the mandala has numbers on it. The professional explains that group member number 1 will color all of the spaces with a 1 inside with their particular color.
4 This continues with group members 2, 3, 4, etc. coloring in their spaces in the mandala that has their number inside. The activity is complete when the mandala is colored by all group members.

Processing and Application: Once the activity has been completed, the professional may ask the group questions, which might include: while looking at the completed mandala, what are your thoughts/feelings about it? Would this picture have looked differently if you had chosen the colors yourself? Completed the activity yourself? How did it feel to work with others in this activity? What do you think about sharing responsibilities? What are other activities where you have to work with others and share responsibilities? Do you think this is important to practice?

Activity: Feelings Collage.
Target Area(s): Expressing and sharing feelings, listening to the feelings of others, and executive functioning.
Level: Adolescents.
Materials: One sheet of paper for each group member, various magazines, scissors, glue, and markers.
Introduction: This activity will allow group members to further explore one feeling of their choosing. Pictures instead of words will be used to describe this feeling. Group members will share their collages and provide feedback to the collages of the other group members.

Instructions:

1 The professional will explain to group members that each person will need to choose a feeling and not share with the other members which feeling they chose (the group can decide if they are o.k. with the chance that the same

feeling is chosen by several group members or not. If not, each group member can whisper in the professional's ear what they chose, and they can let them know if that feeling was chosen already).

2 The professional will give each group member a sheet of paper, and magazines will be available for all. The professional will instruct group members to go through the magazines and tear/cut out any pictures that remind them of their chosen feelings.

3 Once pictures are chosen, the group members will each glue their pictures onto their pieces of paper, creating a collage.

4 When completed, group members can each share their collage, expressing why they chose the pictures, or a feeling-guessing game can be played based on the context of the pictures.

5 Group members can each give feedback to the individual that is presenting, focusing on pictures chosen, presentation, expression of feelings, etc.

Processing and Application: Once every group member has shared, the professional may ask the group additional processing questions, such as: Was it easier or harder to use pictures to describe your feeling? Did you notice any similarities between your chosen pictures and the pictures of other group members? Did any group member share something that you can relate to? How can we use pictures at home/school/etc. to let people know how we're feeling?

Activity: Act As If.
Target Area(s): Handling anxiety and practicing body awareness.
Level: Adolescents.
Materials: None.
Introduction: In therapeutic sessions, we may forget at times to focus on wellness. With this activity, we discuss what it may look like to actually feel the opposite of negative feelings and then use movement to show the positive feelings. This can help group members feel their bodies' responding to positive emotions. They can then take one small action of this expression to practice when feeling dysregulated.

Instructions:

1 The professional brainstorms with group members about what their body feels like when anxious (examples include shaking, head down, mumbling, shoulders hunched, etc.).

2 The professional mimics the suggestions by moving their body as group members have described.

3 The professional then brainstorms with group members what opposite movements would look like. The opposite movement can be whatever the members decide, and the professional can provide some examples.

4 The professional mimics the suggestions by moving their body as group members have described and then invites other group members to walk around the room 'as if' they are not anxious.

Processing and Application: The professional should process with the group members once the activity has been completed. Some sample processing questions include: How did it feel to walk around the room 'as if' you had no anxiety? What is one of the movements you can try to start doing when feeling anxious? Where could moving 'as if' you had no anxiety be helpful?

Activity: Hand Jive.
Target Area(s): Working in a group and cooperation.
Level: Adolescents.
Materials: None.
Introduction: This is a fun way for each group member to use an appropriate hand movement to create a group hand jive. The hand jive can easily be used for an opening or closing transition for subsequent groups. The professional should be prepared for possible inappropriate gestures to be mentioned, and if this happens, calmly explain that the gesture would be inappropriate in a social setting. Other group members can also help explain what could happen if the inappropriate gesture were displayed in various social settings.

Instructions:

1 The professional brainstorms with group members the multiple friendly gestures our hands can do (examples include waving, high-fiving, thumbs up, fist pump, etc.).
2 Each group member chooses the friendly hand gesture that they want to use for the hand jive. It can be a real or made-up gesture, as long as it is not seen as inappropriate or offensive.
3 Once each group member has chosen a hand gesture, the hand jive is created using each gesture from each group member in a continuous movement.
4 Hand jive is practiced multiple times, possibly written down to remember, and can accompany music.

Processing and Application: Once the hand jive activity has been done a few times, the professional may ask the group some processing questions, such as: How can friendly gestures be helpful in social settings? How can unfriendly gestures be unhelpful or possibly offensive in social settings? This activity can assist in opening a discussion about body language – understanding what is meant by body language and how some people communicate through body language.

Activity: I Spy.
Target Area(s): Perspective-taking, recognizing the emotions of others, and communicating feelings to others.
Level: Adolescents.
Materials: A blanket large enough for all group members to sit on.

Introduction: *I Spy* is an excellent intervention to teach parents for their group sessions. It can also be completed with the professional who has access to public areas for viewing. It is important for the parent or professional to have the group members sit at a distance from the public so as not to be overheard while practicing emotion recognition. It is also advisable for the professional or parent to first model how the game is played for greater understanding. Group members may also need to be reminded not to point or yell out during this game; it's strictly a game within the group.

Instructions:

1　The professional or parent brings group members to a public place and has them sit on a blanket an appropriate distance from other people (for example, places including parks, outdoor plazas, etc.).
2　The professional or parent states they are going to play the game *I Spy*. The group members will observe the people around them and propose a feeling they believe a person or other people are feeling. When they believe they have enough context, they can call out, "I spy someone who is feeling _____."
3　Once a group member has called this out, other group members guess which person or people the individual has noticed. Once the correct person has been chosen, group members discuss clues they had to help them guess the feeling.
4　This activity can be played for several minutes, ideally allowing time for each group member to share something they notice.

Processing and Application: Once the activity has been completed, the professional may ask the group questions for further processing. Some example questions include: What did you notice while playing this game? Why do you think we needed to sit away from the public while playing this group? What are clues we noticed about people who were (happy, mad, sad, etc.)? How can this game help you at (school, home, grocery store, etc.)?

Activity: What to Say Scripts.
Target Area(s): Discussing emotions, sharing with a group, and handling difficult situations.
Level: Adolescents.
Materials: Index cards and pencils.
Introduction: Some neurodivergent adolescents may struggle with emotion regulation. When angered by other peers, they may revert to less effective coping methods, such as running away, screaming, hitting themselves, etc. Writing a short script that can be practiced with group members who have struggles can provide an effective means for ensuring success when these difficult situations occur.

Instructions:

1 The professional begins by describing how all of us struggle with what to say when someone upsets us. Having a short phrase written and practiced can often be a useful tool in helping us stay calm when angered (the professional may wish to share an example to help lessen the discomfort with sharing).

2 The professional asks the group member to share something that has been said to them that has made them upset. If the group seems less inclined to share personal anecdotes, the professional can instead ask what things might make adolescents their age upset.

3 Once a group member has spoken, the professional asks other group members to share ideas of a brief phrase that may be an effective coping statement for that situation. The professional should be ready to give an example to help with the group discussion or even have common coping phrases/mantras available for viewing.

4 The group member who shared first then chooses one phrase they wish to use as their coping statement and writes it on their index card. Steps 2–4 continue until every group member has completed this activity.

5 The remaining session time is spent with the group members getting into pairs and practicing using their coping statements. They may choose to practice the statement without the other group member saying the hurtful phrase if it causes too much dysregulation; however, the goal is for the participants to be able to hear the statement in practice to help gain confidence with their response.

6 The professional should encourage this to be practiced multiple times at home so the group members are prepared if/when they encounter the hurtful statement.

Processing and Application: The professional may provide some processing directives at the end of this activity. Describe the bravery it took for you to share with the group something that upsets you. Discuss the feelings you felt when recounting the statement that upset you. Discuss the feelings you felt when the other group members were helping you with helpful coping statements.

Activity: Safe Zones.
Target Area(s): Identifying places to feel safe, recognizing the need for strategies, and working in a group.
Level: Adolescents.
Materials: Graph paper, pencils, and small red, yellow, and green dot stickers.
Introduction: There are many places where neurodivergent adolescents may feel overwhelmed and anxious. Discussing this while also coming up with safe zones within these places can empower clients to feel more comfortable when being in these places. Group members will also discover that they are not alone in feeling this dysregulation, which may normalize their feelings of anxiety.

Instructions:

1 The professional begins by expressing how certain places can make us feel anxious. Examples might include schools, grocery stores, churches, etc.
2 The professional invites the group members to share a place that makes them feel anxious, uncomfortable, or dysregulated.
3 Once group members share, the professional hands each adolescent a piece of graph paper and a pencil. The professional invites the group members to each draw a simple floor plan of the place that causes anxiety. The professional may have a simple sketch drawn already for reference. Listing the rooms and areas within the place would also be helpful for the group members to do.
4 Once completed, the professional asks each group member to look at their drawings and think about where within this place it may be possible to feel calmer or more regulated. Where within this place may they be able to use their coping skills in a safer, acceptable, more private space? The professional hands each group member a sheet containing green, yellow, and red stickers dots. The professional has the members mark safe places with a green dot (consider a floorplan of a school, for example, green spaces may include a special education room, a nurse's office, a counselor's office, etc.).
5 The professional then has the group members mark with a red dot those spaces within the floor plan where it would not feel safe, acceptable, or private to calm down and regulate (using the school example, red spaces may include a music room, a gym, or a playground).
6 The professional then has the group members mark with a yellow dot those spaces within the floor plan where they are not sure if it would feel safe, acceptable, or private to calm down and regulate. They would need to talk to an adult and explore if this space was an option. These areas would be marked with a yellow dot (using the school example, yellow spaces may include a classroom, the office, etc.).
7 Each group member can share and discuss their floorplans with the rest of the group.

Processing and Application: The professional may ask the group processing questions at the end of this activity. A lot of processing has occurred during this activity, so this part may be brief and only focus on a plan of how they can incorporate their floorplan into action.

Activity: Oops and Ouch.
Target Area(s): Expressing feelings and perspective-taking.
Level: Adolescents.
Materials: Two index cards for each group member, one with the word "Oops!" on it; one with the word "Ouch!" on it, the "Oops!" script and "Ouch!" script (for example, scripts at the end of this activity description).

Introduction: Some neurodivergent adolescents can be very honest and can un-intentionally hurt others' feelings with this honesty. They can also feel hurt by what others say to them but are unable to express these hurt feelings. This activity helps group members begin to recognize when they may be hurting someone's feelings and express when their own feelings are being hurt. This activity is excellent for practicing at home, and the professional may want to give group members extra index cards for the entire family to use.

Instructions:

1 The professional gives each group member two index cards; one card has the word "Oops!" on it; the other has the word "Ouch!" on it.

2 The professional begins the dialogue by discussing how sometimes we may say something that hurts someone's feelings and not even know it. The professional may give an example and then invite other group members to share examples.

3 The professional next begins discussion on how sometimes we may have our feelings hurt and not be sure how to let that person know. They may give an example and then invite other group members to share examples.

4 The professional then explains that the "Oops!" and "Ouch!" cards are going to help them begin to explore how to let people know that their feelings have been hurt as well as how they may have hurt others' feelings.

5 The professional explains the "Oops!" card is used whenever a person realizes they may have said something insulting. When this happens, the person talking should stop, hold up the card, and say, "Oops!" This gives the other person a chance to share if their feelings were hurt or if they were not.

6 The professional then explains the "Ouch!" card is used whenever a person is hurt by what someone has said to them. When this happens, the person holds up the card and says "Ouch!" This gives the talker a chance to stop talking, ask for clarification, and apologize if needed.

7 The professional first has two group members read the "Oops!" script aloud. The professional tells the other group members to hold up the "Oops!" card and say, "Oops!" whenever they feel one of the characters may be saying something hurtful or inappropriate. Whenever any group member does this, the professional should stop the reading and have a discussion on which character may have been hurtful, what they said that was hurtful, and what they could have possibly said instead.

8 The professional then has two other group members read the "Ouch!" script aloud. The professional tells the other group members to hold up the "Ouch!" card and say "Ouch!" whenever they feel one of the characters may have hurt feelings. Whenever any group member does this, the professional should stop the reading and have a discussion on which character may have hurt feelings, what was said that made his feelings hurt, and what he could possibly say to the other character.

Processing and Application: The professional may ask the group questions at the end of this activity, including: Can we think of an example where something we said may have hurt someone else's feelings? How can we start noticing this so we aren't hurting people's feelings? Can we think of an example where something that was said to us hurt our feelings? How can we start letting people know they have hurt our feelings? Did all of us agree on what were "Oops!" statements and what were "Ouch!" statements when we heard the stories? What could that be telling us about each other?

Sample "Oops" Script (Group members are listening for when the speaker may need to stop what they are saying because they may be speaking hurtfully).

Jamie: "Hi Jackie, how are you?"
Jackie: "I'm doing great Jamie!"
Jamie: "Do you want to play basketball with me? We can take turns trying to throw the ball into the net."
Jackie: "Sounds great, let's do it!"
Jamie: "I'll throw the ball first, because I'm much better than you. You can watch me and then learn how to be better."
Jackie: "Oh."
Jamie: "Oh man, I missed it, the ball didn't go in like I thought!"
Jackie: "Ha! Ha! You're not as good as you think!"
Jamie: "I guess not!"
Jackie: "Woo Hoo! I got that one in! Yes!"
Jamie: "Nice job!"
Jackie: "Thanks!"
Jamie: "I'm surprised you got it in, you're usually really bad at this."
Jackie: "Am I?"
Jamie: "Yes, I watched you play, and you are usually terrible at basketball."
Jackie: "Well, at least I am a genius at math where you are really, really bad at multiplication."
Jamie: "Oh, that's my mom calling me, I better go inside! See you later Jackie!"
Jackie: "See you later Jamie!"

Sample "Ouch!" Script (Group members are listening for when the listener may be feeling hurt because of what is being said to them).

Antwan: "Hi Marcus, what are you doing right now?"
Marcus: "What does it look like I'm doing?"
Antwan: "I don't know, that's why I asked."
Marcus: "I'm trying to build a Lego tower, only using yellow Legos."
Antwan: "That's really dumb, I hate the color yellow."
Marcus: "Whatever, Antwan. Do you want to help me build it?"

Antwan:	"Sure, but do I have to only use yellow Legos?"
Marcus:	"No, just pick your favorite color and we can have a two-color tower."
Antwan:	"O.K."
Marcus:	"What are you doing? That looks horrible!"
Antwan:	"I'm just adding a landing over here, I think it looks cool."
Marcus:	"I guess that's ok."
Antwan:	"It's definitely o.k. because your tower was boring and plain, so I needed to make it look better."
Marcus:	"Well it doesn't look better, it looks worse, so you aren't helpful at all."
Antwan:	"I'm just going to build my own tower next to yours."
Marcus:	"That's a good idea, then we can have two towers!"
Antwan:	"Maybe later we can build a parking lot with some cars."
Marcus:	"Maybe, but let's just do our towers right now."

Activity: Architects.

Target Area(s): Working together, compromising, and executive functioning.

Level: Adolescents.

Materials: Duct tape, newspaper, yarn, straws, and scissors.

Introduction: This activity can be completed with all of the group members working together or by dividing the group members into teams of two or three. This is up to the professional based on how well the group members can work in teams. *Architects* is a fun way to work on team building while creating a structure of their choice. Having free reign has a team on deciding what to create can cause some differences of opinion. This gives the group members the opportunity to practice compromise and decision-making. The professional may need to give reminders of the importance of working as a team when completing this activity.

Instructions:

1 The professional gives group members a roll of duct tape, a ball of yarn, some newspaper, straws, and scissors (if dividing the group into smaller teams, each team will need these items).
2 The professional explains that the team will create whatever structure they want using only these four items (the scissors are used for cutting only).
3 The professional tells the group to first discuss with each other possible items to build. Once the group comes to a consensus on what should be built, they can then start the construction.
4 The professional gives the group 20 minutes to create their structure, monitoring the group for turn-taking, compromise, and teamwork.

Processing and Application: Once the group members are finished creating their structure. The professional can make comments about what they observed and ask the group some processing questions. What was easy about working as a team? What was difficult about working as a team? Did the structure turn out as you thought it would – how so or not? Did you have to compromise in the group – how so? What were the benefits of working as a team to complete this activity?

Activity: Communication Blocks.
Target Area(s): Communication, listening, executive functioning, working together to complete a task, and perspective-taking.
Level: Adolescents.
Materials: Two matching sets of blocks or Legos.
Introduction: This activity is designed to help adolescents work on improving their ability to communicate when interacting with another person. It also develops perspective-taking. The participants work in pairs while the professional observes and can better assess the components the adolescents might be struggling with. Blocks, Legos, or pictures can be used in this activity, and it can be repeated many times if warranted. Wood or foam blocks can be used, Legos, or a picture can be drawn. This activity will highlight communication and executive functioning and is a good activity to do early in the group meetings and possibly again toward the end of the group meetings to note differences.

Instructions:

1   The professional tells the participants they are going to be working on an activity called communication blocks (or Legos, or pictures). The professional has the group members get into pairs, sitting with their backs to each other.
2   The professional gives both members in the pair a matching set of blocks, so each person has the same blocks in front of them.
3   One person in the pair is designated the instructor, and the other is designated the listener (builder). The instructor builds something with their blocks. Once they are finished, they are going to tell the listener to build the same thing, giving them instructions on exactly what to build without being able to see what the instructor built (remember their backs are to each other the whole time). The instructor tries to give detailed instructions, and the listener can ask questions, with the goal being that both builds come out identical.
4   Once the pair feels like they are finished, they can turn around and see what each other built.
5   If there is time, the activity can be repeated with the pair switching roles.
6   While the activity is being done, the professional should be walking around the room and observing each pair in the process. The professional might want to take notes on communication style, frustration tolerance, and any other things they may notice and want to mention during the processing time.

Processing and Application: Once everyone has finished, they can stay in their pairs for processing time. Each pair can share how their builds came out.

The professional should ask the group how it felt to be in this process, what was challenging, and if anything felt easy. The professional should also address any notes they took while observing each pair in the building process. This is a good time to talk about the strengths observed and suggestions for completing the task. If there is time, the activity can be repeated or the activity can be implemented again in a later group meeting.

Activity: Follow the Leader.
Target Area(s): Following instructions, listening, attention, and regulation.
Level: Adolescents.
Materials: None.
Introduction: *Follow the Leader* is a fun and silly activity that helps adolescents with executive functioning needs and participating in an activity together. It is completed as a whole group exercise and can have many elements added to the activity. It does require some space to move around; it would be challenging to complete this activity in a small room. Because it is a highly playful activity, it could be implemented in an early group session to help participants feel more relaxed.

Instructions:

1 The professional explains they will be doing an activity called *Follow the Leader*.
2 The professional has all the members stand up and get into a line, one behind the other but giving each other some space.
3 The professional explains they will be at the front of the line and will lead the line around the room while giving out instructions for what the line needs to do. The professional will make different moves or actions and the rest of the line must mimic the professional. For example, the professional will start walking and everyone else starts walking (in line), and then the professional might start waving their hands in the air while they are walking – the line would start waving their hands in the air while walking. Anything the professional does, the rest of the line does, and the professional keeps the line walking around the room while doing different moves.
4 Some examples of moves to do in the line include waving hands in the air, making a sound, clapping hands, stomping feet, doing a right or left leg kick out, flapping hands, putting hands on top of your head, hopping, laughing, walking on tippy toes, dancing, acting like you are a plane, spinning around, acting like you are playing a video game, acting like you are driving a car, etc. Anything the professional can think of, they can do. It's important to keep it fun and silly so the participants can enjoy the experience.
5 After the professional has led the line for a few minutes, the professional should ask if any of the participants want to be the leader. The professional should let each of the members be the leader if they want, but no one should be forced to be the leader if they are uncomfortable.

Processing and Application: Once the activity has been completed (which should be no longer than 15–20 minutes), the professional has the group sit in a circle for processing time. The professional should ask the members how it felt to participate in this activity. Additional processing questions might include what was your favorite part of this activity, was there anything you did not like or felt uncomfortable, and if you were a leader, how did it feel to be the leader?

Activity: Play-Doh Relax.
Target Area(s): Executive functioning, listening, regulation, and relaxation.
Level: Adolescents.
Materials: Play-Doh (one for each participant).
Introduction: This activity simultaneously works on executive functioning needs and completing a task sequence while working on interpersonal skills such as regulation, coping skills, and relaxation. Each participant has their own Play-Doh (it is recommended to have the normal size, not the small size bottles). If any members have a sensitivity to Play-Doh, then this activity would not be implemented.

Instructions:

1 The professional passes out a Play-Doh to each group member. If the professional has several colors, the participants can choose their own color.
2 The professional explains they are going to take the group through a series of activities they will be doing with the Play-Doh.
3 The group members can take out their Play-Doh and begin to manipulate it in their hands.
4 The professional then begins to provide instructions for what to do with the Play-Doh. The following guide can be used, or the professional can create their own version.

a Role the Play-Doh into a ball in your hands.
b Squeeze the Play-Doh in your left hand.
c Role the Play-Doh into a snake between your hands.
d Cut or pinch the Play-Doh off into seven pieces.
e Roll the Play-Doh into a ball between your hands.
f Squeeze the Play-Doh in your right hand.
g Using your palms, smash the Play-Doh into a thin layer.
h Make a fist with your left hand, take the Play-Doh, and cover your fist, pressing it down to mold it around your left-hand fist.
i Do the same thing to your right hand.
j Finish playing with the Play-Doh as you like or turn it into anything you want.

Processing and Application: Each of the steps in the Play-Doh sequence should last around two minutes. The professional can add steps and actions. The ending allows the participants two minutes to play with the Play-Doh however they like. Once the activity has been completed, the professional should ask the participants some processing questions, such as how did it feel to complete this activity, did you feel relaxed doing this activity, was there any step that you enjoyed more than the others, and was there any step that you did not like? The professional should also discuss completing this activity or a version of this activity at home or other places when the members might feel anxious, worried, or upset. The professional can ask the members if they can think of a situation where they might use the activity to help them in their daily lives.

Activity: Magazine Minute.
Target Area(s): Safety awareness, masking, understanding social context, and body awareness.
Level: Adolescents.
Materials: A variety of magazines.
Introduction: This activity can work on a variety of needs and provides the opportunity to discuss several different social situations. The professional will need to have several magazines available to use for this activity. The professional should look through each magazine to make sure there is no inappropriate content in the magazines. *Magazine Minute* can be played several times and with different instructions. Some examples are provided in the instructions section, but professionals may want to implement their own versions.

Instructions:

1 The professional has several magazines on a table (the magazines should have examples through stories and/or advertisements of people in different situations or people in general).
2 The professional explains that each member can take a couple of magazines, and when the professional says "Go" the participants will have one minute to find an example of a person or people in the magazine that are in some type of social situation.
3 Once the minute is up, each member will share the picture they found and talk about what social situation they believe is happening. They can share what they think the situation is, how people are reacting, feeling, or anything they want to say about what is happening in the picture.
4 The professional can help any member who is struggling to identify what might be happening in the picture, and other group members can add what they think is happening in other members pictures.
5 The professional should then complete the process a couple more times as time permits.

Processing and Application: Once the activity has finished, the professional can have a processing time with the members. Some suggested processing questions include how did it feel completing this activity, what felt challenging to you and what felt easy, did you find pictures that seemed confusing or that you did not understand what was happening, and how does this apply to your daily life when you see people in social situations? This activity can prompt a good discussion about the members' daily lives and confusion or needs in social situations in which they do not understand what is happening or feel challenged in participating. It can also open a good discussion about masking and how and why masking occurs.

Activity: Wall Draw.
Target Area(s): Completing a task together, teamwork, cooperation, paying attention to another person, and communication.
Level: Adolescents.
Materials: Large piece of paper, tape, and markers.
Introduction: *Wall Draw* is a whole group activity. If the group has a large number of members (8–10), this activity should be divided into two groups. This activity gives the group members an opportunity to work together as a team to complete a task. Neurodivergent adolescents may struggle in peer groups, especially when asked to work in a group setting to accomplish something. *Wall Draw* is a fun and relaxed way to help navigate participating in a group. The professional will want to observe each group member and possibly take notes on skill strengths and struggles.

Instructions:

1   The professional explains to the group they will be drawing a picture together. The professional makes sure to state that drawing skills are not necessary to complete this task and the objective is fun – not creating a great drawing.
2   The professional hangs a large piece of paper on the wall or lays it on a table.
3   The professional gives each member a different color marker.
4   The professional decides on the drawing order, giving each participant a number indicating when they will draw on the paper.
5   The professional explains that each member will go in number order to the paper and draw something. Each member will have 20 seconds to draw. When their 20 seconds are up, the next person will go for 20 seconds and draw on the paper. This will continue until each member has drawn on the paper twice. The group members can talk and decide on a unified picture to draw, or they can randomly add to the picture. This will be something the group needs to decide. The professional can provide guidance if needed.
6   Once the picture has been completed, the members can look at the finished product and notice each person's contribution (remember each person will have their own color of marker).
7   All the members can then sign the picture they have created together.

Processing and Application: Once the picture has been completed, the professional asks the group members some processing questions, such as what did it feel like to complete this picture together, was it easy to work together or difficult, what was the easiest part and hardest part for you, and do you think it would have felt better to draw your own picture? The professional can also share any observations they noted while the members were completing the picture. The professional can also ask the members about times in their daily lives when they had to work with a group and what the experience was like.

Activity: Make a Monster.
Target Area(s): Working together, communication, executive functioning, and frustration tolerance.
Level: Adolescents.
Materials: Piece of paper, marker, scissors, and a blindfold (handkerchief or scarf).
Introduction: Some neurodivergent adolescents struggle to interact with their peers, especially with in-person conversation and communication. This activity helps adolescents become more comfortable with communication as well as navigating as a team through a fun and engaging game. Further need targets might include executive functioning and managing frustration tolerance. The professional will do some pre-meeting set-up work with this activity. The professional will draw an outline of a monster on a piece of paper (it should be a large outline). The professional will then cut the monster into puzzle pieces (the number of pieces should match the number of group members). The professional will want to have this ready prior to the group meeting.

Instructions:

1 The professional will explain to the group they will be completing an activity called *Make a Monster*.
2 The professional will give each member a piece of the monster puzzle and explain to the participants that these are pieces of a monster outline.
3 The group must work together to complete the puzzle (make the monster).
4 Each member will take a turn placing their pieces on the table to try and connect to other members' pieces and complete the puzzle. But the person who is putting their piece in play will be blindfolded, and the rest of the group must communicate to that person where to place their puzzle piece.
5 For example, each member takes a turn placing their piece. The person who is going must be blindfolded with a handkerchief or a scarf. The rest of the group guides that person to where they place their piece. They then take off their blindfold, and it is given to the person who goes next. This continues until all the pieces have been placed correctly and the monster has been made.
6 The professional should be observing the interaction among the group members, specifically noting strengths and struggles.

Processing and Application: Once the puzzle has been completed, the professional processes the activity with the group. Some suggested processing questions include how did you feel completing this activity, what was challenging and what was easy, how did it feel to be blindfolded and having to rely on the group members to help you, and what do you feel like you learned from completing this activity? The professional should also share any observations they made while watching the group complete the activity.

Appendix

Step by Step Guide for Implementing AutPlay Groups

1 *Group Structure*: Establish a group meeting location, any support professional that will be working with you to facilitate the group, and what your group fee will be. Decide on the size of the group (this will help determine how many adults need to be involved) and how long the group will meet. This book outline 10 in clinic 50-minute groups but this can vary depending on participant needs, group wants, and billing specifics. All the group structure components can vary greatly and should be decided on by the professional depending on their work setting.

2 *Market the Group*: Establish the age range and type of group member that will be participating, establish this before marketing a group and target the type of group being offered. Also, decide and indicate on marketing materials if it will be a play group or a topic focused group, or possibly both. Otherwise began a general marketing effort and see who signs up and form the group(s) accordingly. Reach out to local agencies and organizations, promote the group online, and let other therapists in the community know about the group.

3 *Meet with the Caregivers and Child*: As people indicate an interest in participating in a group, meet with the caregivers and child. This is a time to get more information about the child and observe the child. The caregiver should complete the Intake Form, Group Readiness Form, Confidentiality Form, Social Navigation Inventory, Play Assessment, and any additional paperwork that is needed. After this meeting and upon review of the completed forms, the professional should make one of the following decisions regarding participation in a group:

   – Sign the child up for a group that is beginning.
   – Place the child on a waiting list for when an appropriate group begins.
   – Discuss with the caregiver that the child may not be ready for a group and offer individual therapy or a referral.

4 *Establish the Schedule*: Once the group members have been selected, complete the group schedule. Establish with the caregivers who will be hosting an outside of the clinic meeting and when this will take place – make sure to indicate these dates on the Group Schedule Form. The caregivers should be given the completed Group Schedule Form before the first group meeting. This schedule will show caregivers when in clinic groups are happening and when a parent hosting meeting is happening. Also, give caregivers the Participants Contact Information Form. This will enable caregivers to contact other caregivers when hosting an outside of the clinic meeting.

5 *First Session*: Begin the first group session in the clinic location. Follow the group meetings guide in this book. Remember this is just a guide, the professional has the flexibility to add, integrate, and adapt from the guide. Once group sessions begin, it is a consistent and organized routine that happens week to week until the 20 meetings (in clinic sessions and out of clinic meetings) have ended.

6 *Session Overview Form*: At the end of each session, the professional should give the caregivers the Session Overview Form. This form highlights what was worked on in the session, how to continue to support group therapy goals at home, and information about the next week's caregiver hosted meeting. The professional should have the form completed before the group begins for easy distribution to all the caregivers at the end of the group meeting.

7 Continue with groups two through ten following the group meetings guide in this book. Again, remember this is a guide and the professional may adapt or integrate protocol throughout the ten meetings as needed. This is something the professional will decide based on what they feel is appropriate and helpful for their groups. AutPlay Groups have an intentional looseness to give professionals the ability to individualize their groups based on their expertise and the needs of the children and adolescents in the group.

8 Group 10 will be the last group meeting and should provide closure for the group. The group meeting guide in this book provides information on terminating the group. Professionals should consider if it would be beneficial for a group to continue to meet. In some cases, ten meetings will not be enough for a child or adolescent to achieve their therapy goals. The professional could decide to continue the group for an additional set number of sessions, continue the group indefinitely, start another group with some previous group participants and some new participants.

AutPlay Groups Sample Marketing Letter

Date:

Dear Parent/Caregiver of _____:

Hello. My name is _____, and I am beginning an AutPlay Group. AutPlay Therapy is a neurodiversity informed and affirming collaborative process designed to value the individual child and highlight their strengths as well as guide areas of intervention, goals, and approaches for addressing the needs of the child and family. It is a neurodiversity-affirming framework for implementing play therapy. The AutPlay framework is neurodiversity paradigm informed and designed to help child and play therapists address the mental health needs of neurodivergent children ages 3–18 (autistic children, those with ADHD, social anxiety, sensory differences, learning differences, and developmental and physical disabilities). The AutPlay Group will work on (fill in the blank).

This group will meet weekly on _____ at _____.
In addition to in-clinic sessions, there will also be weekly groups hosted by each caregiver. This is a fun and informative way for the group members to further connect, while caregivers can get to know each other and learn more about how to facilitate interaction with their child. There will also be ideas given to caregivers on how to support therapy goals at home.

Please complete the form below if you are interested in your child attending this group. I will need the form returned to me by _____.

Thank you for your interest!

Sincerely,

_____ cut here _____

I give permission for my child, _____, to attend the AutPlay Group. I understand this group meets in-clinic weekly and will also have caregiver hosted meetings. I am willing to host one of these groups.

_____   _____
Caregiver Signature   Date

Caregiver Contact Information

_____

_____

AutPlay Groups Intake Form Page One

Name: _____ Date of Birth: _____

Parent(s)/Caregiver(s) Name(s): _____

Address: _____
          Street number and name   City   State   Zip Code

Phone Number: (___)_____ Okay to leave a message? Yes or No (circle one)

Email Address: _____

In Case of Emergency Notify: _____ Phone: (___) _____

Primary Care Physician: _____ Phone: (___) _____

List any and all diagnosis your child has received: _____
_____

List any medical problems that I need to be aware of: _____
_____

List all medications that are currently being prescribed: _____
_____

List any allergies, including food allergies/sensitivities: _____
_____

Does your child have any sensory processing differences: _____
_____

Describe your child's social navigation: _____
_____
_____
_____
_____

Describe your child's play preferences and strengths: _____
_____
_____
_____
_____

AutPlay Groups Intake Form Page Two

Fee and Payment Information

Fees for group sessions are due and payable on the day of service unless other arrangements are made prior to the time of service. Cash, credit card, and checks are accepted. Many insurance plans are accepted. Clients should consult their insurance provider for information regarding co-payment, deductible, and number of authorized sessions. Regardless of what an insurance company states to this office or you about payment for services, this is not a guarantee of payment for services. You are still responsible for full payment for group services even if an insurance company states they will pay and do not.

Co-pays must be paid at the time of the session. If the office must mail you an invoice, then a processing fee of $_____ will be applied. Co-pays can be paid to the front office staff or your therapist. A copy of your insurance card should be on file with this office.

Medicaid and MC+ are accepted. A copy of the Medicaid or MC+ card should be on file with this office. The average group session time lasts one hour. The standard fee per group session is $_____.

Medicaid

Name of Child on Medicaid Card:_____

Medicaid Number:_____ Birth Date: _____

Private Insurance

Name of Responsible Party on Insurance Card: _____

Parent Social Security # _____ Child Social Security # _____

Insurance Company/Plan: _____

Individual #_____ Group #_____

Insurance Company Billing Address & Phone Number: _____

_____

_____

I have read and understood the above related fee payment information and agree to the terms defined by this office.

_____   _____   _____
Client Name   Caregiver Signature   Date

AutPlay Groups Intake Form Page Three

Cancelation of Sessions and No-Show Sessions

If a group meeting is scheduled and needs to be canceled, you must cancel by phone prior to the scheduled group meeting time. If you fail to cancel before the scheduled group meeting time, you will be charged a $_____ fee that must be paid before continuing with sessions. Further, if a group meeting is missed with no cancelation made, you are not guaranteed a continued spot in the group. It is your responsibility to contact this office if a group meeting needs to be canceled and to verify any future group meetings. Exceptions to these guidelines include a crisis situation, emergency, disaster, or unexpected illness.

Record Requests and Release

Minimal records are kept regarding group meetings, but basic intake, consent, and session notes are maintained. You may ask to see your child's records or request a copy of your child's records at any time. We do require a seven-day notice for a records request. You may also request a report be written to a third party at any time. Requests for a report of any type must be given at least seven days in advance. We cannot guarantee any request for a report that has been submitted with less than a seven-day notice - the report will likely not be provided by the requested date. Please note that when requesting a specific report be written, a reasonable fee will be charged for providing a copy of your report or a summary of records which would include cost of copying, postage, and preparation or an explanation or summary of the information.

Court Related Records, Testimony, and Appearance

If the therapist is requested or subpoenaed at any point in time to appear in court or participate in court related activities on you or your child's behalf, you will be responsible for payment reimbursement of the therapist's time which will be billed at a rate of $_____ per hour. Travel time spent to and from court or other venues related to court activities will be considered part of the hourly time billed. If records or documents are requested or subpoenaed, a reasonable fee will be charged for providing a copy of your records or a summary of those records which would include cost of copying, postage, and preparation or an explanation or summary of the information.

I have read and understood the above related fee payment information and court related information and agree to the terms defined by this office.

_____   _____   _____
Client Name   Caregiver Signature   Date

AutPlay Groups Confidentiality Statement

All persons participating in group therapy must read and sign this agreement. If you do not understand any part of this agreement, please ask any questions prior to signing the agreement.

Confidentiality:

Anything said between group members at any time is part of the group and is confidential. I understand that everything said in this group is confidential and not to be shared with anyone outside of the group, except as may be otherwise required by law. I understand this includes in clinic group meetings as well as caregiver hosted outside clinic group meetings and play times.

- I agree to keep confidential the names of other members of the group and what is said in the group. As a member of this group, I agree to not disclose to anyone outside the group any information that may identify another group member. This includes, but is not limited to, names, physical descriptions, biological information, and specifics to the content of interactions with other group members.
- I agree to indemnify and hold _____ harmless for any loss or damages, including costs and attorney's fees, incurred by _____ as a result of my breach of another's confidentiality.

I also understand that anything said in group therapy is confidential, *except* for the following limitations:

- Child abuse and/or neglect.
- Vulnerable adult abuse or neglect.
- Threats to harm oneself.
- Threats regarding harm to another person.
- A court subpoena.
- My specific request, in writing, to disclose information regarding my psychotherapy to a third party.

Please note that if you choose to send communications through text or email these communications are not protected and confidentiality cannot be assured.

By my signature below, I indicate that I have read carefully and understand the AutPlay Groups Confidentiality Statement and I agree to its terms and conditions. I am aware signing the Agreement is required for my admission to the group. I am also aware that my refusal to sign this Agreement will exclude me from participating in the group.

Caregiver/Client Name (print): _____

Guardian Signature: _____

Date: _____

AutPlay Group Readiness Questionnaire - Page One

Child Name _____ Age _____

Caregiver(s) Name _____ Phone _____

What diagnosis (if any) does your child have?

Does your child have any physical disabilities or physical needs? Does your child need any accommodations to participate in a therapy group?

Describe your child's social interaction and play preferences.

Describe your child's communication style and preferences.

Has your child ever participated in a therapy or play group before? If so, what was the experience like for your child?

What does your child like to do for fun?

What are some of your child's interests?

What community/public activities has your child participated in that they seemed to enjoy?

What community/public activities has your child participated in that they seemed to not enjoy?

What seems to help your child regulate, calm, or relax?

AutPlay Group Readiness Questionnaire - Page Two

Child Name_____ Age _____

Parent(s) Name _____ Phone _____

What sensory differences (if any) does your child seem to respond negatively to (large crowds, noise, etc.)?

What would you like to see improve for your child by participating in this group?

What do you feel would be your child's biggest challenge with participating in this group?

Would your child do well with older children, younger children, children of the opposite gender?

How would you like this group to assist you as a caregiver?

Are you willing to participate in the group experience with your child?

Any additional information you would like to share with us about your child?

AutPlay Groups Participants Contact Information

Child's Name _____

Caregiver's Name and Contact Information _____

_____

Child's Name _____

Caregiver's Name and Contact Information _____

_____

Child's Name _____

Caregiver's Name and Contact Information _____

_____

Child's Name _____

Caregiver's Name and Contact Information _____

_____

Child's Name _____

Caregiver's Name and Contact Information _____

_____

Child's Name _____

Caregiver's Name and Contact Information _____

_____

Child's Name _____

Caregiver's Name and Contact Information _____

_____

Child's Name _____

Caregiver's Name and Contact Information _____

_____

Child's Name _____

Caregiver's Name and Contact Information _____

_____

AutPlay Groups Schedule

	Clinic or Caregiver Hosted (Circle One)	Date	Time	Additional Information
Week One	Clinic caregiver			
Week Two	Clinic caregiver			
Week Three	Clinic caregiver			
Week Four	Clinic caregiver			
Week Five	Clinic caregiver			
Week Six	Clinic caregiver			
Week Seven	Clinic caregiver			
Week Eight	Clinic caregiver			
Week Nine	Clinic caregiver			
Week Ten	Clinic caregiver			
Week Eleven	Clinic caregiver			
Week Twelve	Clinic caregiver			
Week Thirteen	Clinic caregiver			
Week Fourteen	Clinic caregiver			
Week Fifteen	Clinic caregiver			
Week Sixteen	Clinic caregiver			
Week Seventeen	Clinic caregiver			
Week Eighteen	Clinic caregiver			
Week Nineteen	Clinic caregiver			
Week Twenty	Clinic caregiver			

AutPlay Group Session Overview Form

Date: _____

Group Session Number: _____

Session Summary:

Home Practice:

Additional Information:

Next In-Clinic Session: _____

Next Caregiver Hosting Meeting: _____

- Name of caregiver _____
- Location of event _____

AutPlay Group Session Overview Form - Example

Date: January 25, 2024

Group Session Number: 4

Session Summary: Today's focus was on personal space. We learned how all of us feel comfortable with a different amount of space! It's important to be aware of this, and to ask others if we are giving them enough personal space and tell others we need more space. We can also look for cues that someone is uncomfortable with how close we are to them (they are backing away from us for example).

Home Practice: Practice personal space in a variety of settings. This can be in a line, having a conversation, going down a slide, etc. You can use a prop, such as a piece of string or a pool noodle to discover how much personal space each family member needs. You can also come up with a special word when you feel you need more space (a word as simple as 'Space') and practice using this word as a family.

Additional Information: Personal space can be a difficult concept, so practice it often. Once learned, repeated practice may be needed in a variety of other sessions.

Next In-Clinic Session: February 8, 2024 at 10:00 a.m.
Next Caregiver Hosting Session: February 1, 2024 at 10:00 a.m.

- Name of caregiver: Janice Jackson
- Location of event: Hubert Park, 123 Main Street

AutPlay Groups Caregiver Update Form

Please complete this form and provide information about your child's experience and participation in outside of the clinic caregiver hosted meetings.

Caregiver's Name: _____

Child's Name: _____

Describe the Activity in Which your Child Participated:

Describe any Observations About your Child's Participation:

Describe any Challenges or Issues you Noticed:

Describe any Strengths or Positives you Noticed:

AutPlay Groups Session Note

Child's Name_____ Date_____

Group Meeting # _____ Time _____ Group Procedure Code _____

Child' Diagnosis _____ Group Facilitator _____

Group Members Present _____

_____

_____

_____

Group Intervention, Approach, or Activity (as related to therapy goals):

_____

Child's Response to Group Participation:

_____

Child's Progress in Group (as related to therapy goals):

_____

Additional Information:

_____   _____

Signature of Professional   Date

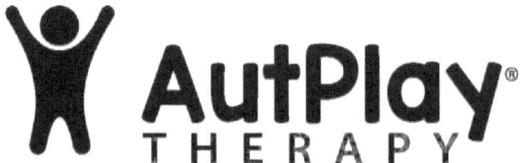

AutPlay® Group
Certificate of Completion

This completion certificate is awarded to

Child Name

_____

Caregiver Name

_____

For successfully completing the AutPlay Group experience.

Signature of Facilitator   Date

_____

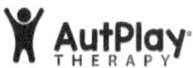

AutPlay® Assessment of Play – Page One

Child's Name_____Age_____Gender_____Date_____

Read the following play categories and definitions and rate where you feel your child is at in terms of possessing and demonstrating this type of play.

Functional Play is a term also used for relational play, it means denoting use of objects in play for the purposes for which they were intended, e.g., using simple objects correctly, combining related objects, and making objects do what they are made to do (setting up a bowling set and bowling).
NO - 1   2   3   4   5   6   7   8   9   10   - YES

Symbolic Play refers to symbolic, or pretend play which occurs when children begin to substitute one object for another. For example, using a hairbrush to represent a microphone. The child may pretend to do something (with or without the object present or with an object representing another object) or be someone.
NO - 1   2   3   4   5   6   7   8   9   10   - YES

Cooperative Play refers to a play where children plan, assign roles, and play together. Cooperative play is goal-oriented and children play in an organized manner toward a common end. Moreover, Cooperative play is a "true social play" in which children cooperate or assume reciprocal roles.
NO - 1   2   3   4   5   6   7   8   9   10   - YES

Sociodramatic Play refers to play involving acting out scripts, scenes, and plays adopted from cartoons, books. Children take/assume roles using themselves and/or characters like dolls, figures, and puppets as they interact together on common themes.
NO - 1   2   3   4   5   6   7   8   9   10   - YES

Peer play refers to interactions with one's peers, which provide opportunities for physical, cognitive, social, and emotional development.
NO - 1   2   3   4   5   6   7   8   9   10   - YES

Constructive Play characterized as manipulation of objects for the purpose of constructing or creating something. Children use materials to achieve a specific goal in mind that requires transformation of objects into a new configuration. Lego pieces turned to cars or houses are an example of this play.
NO - 1   2   3   4   5   6   7   8   9   10   - YES

Sensory Play involves playing with toys or items for the purpose of sensory sensations or sensory seeking. Enjoying the toy or object because of how it feels or what it produces for the senses. Sensory balls, putty, and exercise balls are examples.

NO - 1   2   3   4   5   6   7   8   9   10   - YES

Technology Play characterized by playing online and video games alone or with others. This might involve a tablet, a game station, or playing games on a computer.

NO - 1   2   3   4   5   6   7   8   9   10   - YES

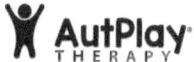

AutPlay® Assessment of Play – Page Two

Child's Name_____Age_____Gender_____Date_____

Please answer the following questions regarding your child's play. Try to think about specific times you have observed or played with your child and answer the questions as completely as possible.

Does your child play with toys?

Does your child play independently?

Does your child play with other children?

Does your child initiate play with other children or adults?

Do you have play times with your child?

Does your child interact with you during play times?

Does your child do pretend play or metaphor play?

Does your child play with objects that would not be considered toys?

If someone (child or adult) asks your child to play, what does your child usually do?

Does your child seem to want to play?

Does your child seem to like technology-based play?

Describe your child's play.

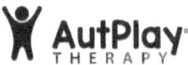

AutPlay® Social Navigation Inventory

Name _____**Age____Gender ____ Date _____**

How would you describe your child's social navigation?

_____

_____

_____

Does your child play with or hang out with others? Please describe.

_____

_____

_____

Please describe any of the following possible needs your child may be having–experiencing bulling, peer rejection, safety awareness concerns, social anxiety, misunderstood by others, self-esteem struggles, self-awareness issues, unhappy with current peer/friendship situations.

_____

_____

_____

What is your child's social and other strengths?

_____

_____

_____

What does social navigation look like in your family?

_____

_____

_____

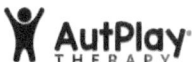

AutPlay® Groups Neurodiversity-Affirming Guide

(eight questions for professionals to complete)

1 Do I understand what neurodiversity-affirming means? How am I being affirming in this approach or intervention?

2 Have I assessed the method or protocol I'm using to make sure it is affirming?

3 When focusing on social navigation, does working on the social need help the child better get what they want?

4 When working on social navigation, does working on the social need address an issue/struggle the child is having?

5 When working on social navigation, have I considered if there is really a child's need or is it a socially expected neurotypical standard the child is being held to?

6 When working on social navigation, have I considered the "problem" is not the child, but an adult the child is encountering or an environment?

7 Is the child being given a voice to communicate what they think, feel, and want?

8 Does the therapeutic process implemented consistently stay affirming for the child and are differences and preferences being valued and not labeled as needs?

Feelings List

Accepted	Afraid	Affectionate	Loyal
Angry	Miserable	Anxious	Misunderstood
Peaceful	Beautiful	Playful	Ashamed
Brave	Awkward	Calm	Proud
Capable	Quite	Bored	Overwhelmed
Caring	Relaxed	Confused	Cheerful
Relieved	Defeated	Comfortable	Safe
Competent	Satisfied	Concerned	Mad
Depressed	Pressured	Confident	Provoked
Content	Desperate	Regretful	Courageous
Silly	Lonely	Rejected	Curious
Special	Disappointed	Remorseful	Strong
Discouraged	Disgusted	Sad	Sympathetic
Excited	Embarrassed	Shy	Forgiving
Thankful	Sorry	Friendly	Thrilled
Fearful	Stubborn	Nervous	Stupid
Glad	Understood	Frustrated	Good
Unique	Furious	Tired	Grateful
Valuable	Guilty	Touchy	Great
Hateful	Happy	Helpless	Hopeful
Wonderful	Hopeless	Humorous	Worthwhile
Unattractive	Joyful	Uncertain	Lovable
Humiliated	Uncomfortable	Loved	Hurt
Ignored	Impatient	Indecisive	Inferior
Insecure	Irritated	Jealous	Worried

Neurodivergent Social Navigation List

Explore the list of social navigation components and place a check by any that you feel is a need area for your child. Also, feel free to complete one for yourself on things you may want to better understand.

☐ Recognizing Bullying	☐ Asking for Help
☐ Handling Bullying	☐ Communicating Needs
☐ Self Relaxation Techniques	☐ Standing up for Self and Others
☐ Self-Advocacy	☐ Safety Awareness
☐ Asking Questions	☐ Problem Solving
☐ Regulation Ability	☐ Emotion Awareness
☐ Strengths Awareness	☐ Self Worth
☐ Decision Making	☐ Frustration Tolerance
☐ Personal Space	☐ Styles of Humor
☐ Initiating a Task	☐ Completing a Task
☐ Navigating Groups	☐ Friendship Expectations
☐ Perspective Taking	☐ Self-Compassion
☐ Addressing Anxiety	☐ Understanding Stimming
☐ Sensory Awareness/needs	☐ Executive Functioning Needs
☐ Modulating Emotions	☐ Self-Compassion
☐ Understanding Neurodivergent Differences	☐ Receiving Feedback
☐ Awareness of Rejection Sensitive Dysphoria	☐ Understanding Ableism
☐ Awareness of Play Preferences	☐ Online Safety (navigation)
☐ Awareness of Social Model of Disability	☐ Awareness of Special Interests
☐ Awareness of the Double Empathy Problem	☐ Awareness of Masking
☐ Awareness of Monotropism	☐ Neurodivergent (Identity) Awareness

☐ Social Pragmatics (stopping at a stop sign, paying for things, waiting in a line, etc.). List below:

Additional Group Resources

Grant, R. J. (2023). *The AutPlay therapy handbook: Integrative family play therapy with neurodivergent children.* Routledge.

Grant, R. J. (2024). *Play interventions for neurodivergent children and adolescents: Promoting growth, empowerment, and affirming practices.* Routledge.

Mellenthin, C., Stone, J., & Grant, R. J. (2022). *Implementing play therapy with groups: Contemporary issues in practice.* Routledge.

Sweeney, D. S., Baggerly, J. N., & Ray, D. C. (2014). *Group play therapy: A dynamic approach.* Routledge.

Sweeney, D. S., & Homeyer, L. (1999). *Handbook of group play therapy: How to do it, how it works, whom it's best for.* Jossey-Bass.

Index

Note: **Bold** page numbers refer to tables.